Medical Presentations

This book will teach healthcare professionals how to craft more effective and engaging PowerPoint® presentations, taking readers through the preparation of a presentation from concept to delivery. The book is based on decades of the authors' personal experiences teaching PowerPoint® and slide design. The text is based on a sound understanding of educational theory. Readers will learn how to present interesting and visually appealing slides. In particular, the focus will be on designing professional-looking slides that convey a clear and memorable message.

The book will be valuable to any healthcare professional required to put together presentations, whether a high-flying academic doctor or nurse presenting their research at international conferences, a trainee giving a talk at an in-house educational session or a student preparing a presentation as part of their course work.

T0260421

Medical Presentations
A Prescription for Success

Terry Irwin, Julie Terberg, and Echo Swinford

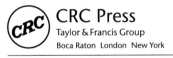

CRC Press
Taylor & Francis Group
Boca Raton London New York

CRC Press is an imprint of the
Taylor & Francis Group, an **informa** business

Designed cover image: gettyimages-855597368-170667a

First edition published 2024
by CRC Press
2385 NW Executive Center Drive, Suite 320, Boca Raton FL 33431

and by CRC Press
4 Park Square, Milton Park, Abingdon, Oxon, OX14 4RN

CRC Press is an imprint of Taylor & Francis Group, LLC

ISBN: 9781032263540 (hbk)
ISBN: 9781032263526 (pbk)
ISBN: 9781003287902 (ebk)

DOI: 10.1201/9781003287902

Typeset in Minion
by KnowledgeWorks Global Ltd.

Contents

Foreword by Professor Trisha Greenhalgh

The best lecture I ever attended was called "How to give a lecture" by Professor Lewis Elton. Elton (yes, Ben's dad) was a distinguished physicist before he became gripped with the problem of student disengagement and underperformance in universities and retrained as a professor of higher education.

The first ten minutes of his lecture consisted of what might be called death by bullet points. Elton (already in his 80s and looking every inch the eccentric, tatty-jacketed old don) falteringly opened a PowerPoint presentation, which crashed and had to be re-booted, and then proceeded to show dull clip art and read off blocks of text in a monotone.

But then he stopped, turned off the computer, removed his jacket, rolled up his sleeves and invited the audience to help him fill a flip chart with all his mistakes. Everything on the list, including the technology crash, along with numerous additional slip-ups they'd failed consciously to notice (such as his scruffy attire and a faltering manner which raised the unconscious suspicion that the old don might be losing his marbles), had been carefully planned to illustrate pedagogical and presentational points. See Chapter 18 for more examples. He then gave a much better PowerPoint presentation illustrating all the points he'd already drawn out on the flip chart.

Elton's key point: the potential for PowerPoint to make a bad presentation even worse is limitless. His bottom line: Learn how students learn—and use the technology accordingly. One of his better slides consisted of a cartoon of a suited lecturer speaking confidently to a packed lecture theatre of blank faces. The speech bubble says: "I am talking and you are listening. Because I am talking and you are not, ideas must be passing from my mouth into your heads. You are being educated.". Nothing, of course, is further from the truth.

Like Lewis Elton, Terry Irwin, Julie Terberg and Echo Swinford take cognitive theory as their starting point. We cannot design our presentations optimally if we do not understand how people process the information and ideas we present. Do not skip this first chapter! Unlike Lewis Elton, they are not interested only in educational lectures. We all make and give PowerPoint presentations to impress and influence people (the last one I gave was to a grant funder). What do you want your audience to do as a result of seeing and hearing this presentation? This book is about influence, not just information transfer or student learning.

If you ever use PowerPoint (or similar technologies), it will be worth your while to work carefully through the chapters in this book. Each is perhaps an evening's work. Like Elton, the authors use the trope of showing you a bad example before improving on it. In Chapter 3, for example, they take you through what seems to be a not-too-terrible set of opening slides for a job interview. You then get to imagine what is going through the mind of a member of the interview panel (another set of broadly correct, worthy-but-dull bullet points). And then they show you how to knock the socks off the other candidates with an imaginative, appealing presentation which will achieve the goal of putting you above all the other candidates in the minds of the panel.

Not covered in this book is the sociological literature on how PowerPoint has come to shape, sometimes in sinister ways, what goes on in organisations. See, for example, JoAnn Yates and Wanda Orlikowski's The PowerPoint Presentation and its Corollaries[1] and Yiannis Gabriel's Against the Tyranny of PowerPoint[2]. Of relevance to this book is how PowerPoint has become the de facto means of communication within and between organisations, departments and working groups; its functionality and affordances have created both opportunities and constraints. Organisations have unwritten rules about how audiences should behave during and after such presentations. It follows, sociologically speaking, that if we engage with this technology only passively and uncritically, we will both produce and reproduce the culture of boredom and disengagement that are a significant downside of this genre in many organisations. But if we engage critically and creatively with PowerPoint and other communicative technologies, we can potentially deploy them in radical ways to change organisations in worthwhile directions.

But that, perhaps, is another book—or, at least, an additional chapter for a future edition.

Trisha Greenhalgh
Professor of Primary Care Health Sciences and
Fellow of Green Templeton College at the University of Oxford
Professor of Primary Health Care and Dean for Research Impact
Queen Mary University, London

NOTES

1. Yates, J. and Orlikowski, W., 2007. The PowerPoint presentation and its corollaries: How genres shape communicative action in organizations. *Communicative practices in workplaces and the professions: Cultural perspectives on the regulation of discourse and organizations*, 1, pp. 67–92.
2. Gabriel, Y., 2008. Against the tyranny of PowerPoint: Technology-in-use and technology abuse. *Organization Studies*, 29(2), pp. 255–276.

Foreword by Dame Parveen Kumar

Medical education has changed enormously over the last two decades, both in the content and in the methodology of teaching. However despite these changes, the use of PowerPoint presentations has become ubiquitous! PowerPoint is used in lectures, seminars, and conferences in all jobs, careers and educational institutions throughout the world.

This is perhaps because the program is perceived as easy to use, with a very short learning curve. However we have all been to, and even given, poor presentations, often due to a lack of preparation and poor slide design, leaving the audience bored and uninterested. We may get bogged down in the detail without signposting and often overloading our presentation slides in the enthusiasm of getting all the facts on one slide!

This book gives a practical account of PowerPoint and, interestingly, starts with the educational theory behind a presentation. This sounds odd, but it is important to know the audience and their level of understanding and to be able to convey that "One Big Idea", avoiding cognitive overload so they will remember the point you are making. Preparation is all important.

The appropriate use of PowerPoint presentations can enhance teaching and learning activities. This is where this book fits in well, as it discusses the basics of making slides and the presentation. It describes the preparation, which is crucial, from the choice of a template, the styles and size of fonts, the amount of text and, above all, not overloading with too much information. Emphasis is placed on the concept that pictures say much more than words (and are also more memorable).

This book is self-contained. Chapters discuss how to give a talk, from who the audience is to how you should plan and prepare the talk. It gives useful hints and examples and references to move on if you want to know more. Pictures are often difficult to insert, and the book leads us to how to access them and how to insert them into your presentation without losing definition.

Many of us have moved on to online lecture deliveries since the pandemic. There are helpful points on how to make these more impactful and how to involve the audience online by using useful strategies.

The authors have a depth of knowledge in teaching and design presentation. One is a clinician with many years of teaching experience, and the others are professional presentation designers.

I would recommend this book to everyone who uses PowerPoint as their preferred teaching method. They will find this book an invaluable adjunct for a career in teaching and communication.

Dame Parveen Kumar DBE
Professor of Medicine and Education
Barts and The London School of Medicine and Dentistry
Author of *Kumar and Clarke's Textbook of Medicine*

Acknowledgements

We would like to thank a number of people who have helped us bring this book to fruition. We are grateful to our publisher, Taylor and Francis, particularly Jo Koster, who believed in this adventure from the start.

We are not so grateful to Noah Webster, American lexicographer, who decided that American English spelling was more logical than British English. We have had to decide which side of the pond to base our writing style on, and the UK won on this occasion! Hopefully our American readers will forgive us.

Dr Gareth Lewis, who has partnered with Terry in teaching presentation skills for several years, provided helpful examples of some of the slides. Without his support in the teaching of presentation skills, it is also doubtful whether this book would have seen the light of day.

Many of the lessons in this book are based on real-world problems faced by learners in those courses. We thank the senior doctors and medical students who provided inspiration and, in some cases, allowed us to use their slides, either as they are or as inspiration. Most have asked to remain anonymous so their names do not appear in the text.

Writing a book of this complexity takes time, and this has taken us away from our families. We hope that they will forgive us for this.

About the authors

Between them, the authors of this book have over 75 years of design and teaching experience, principally based on Microsoft® PowerPoint®. Terry and Julie have co-authored a previous book on developing effective presentations, which won the 2005 British Medical Association's prize for best book in the Basis of Medicine category. Julie and Echo have written a widely acclaimed book on PowerPoint templates, now in its second edition.

Terry Irwin is a retired consultant surgeon based in the UK. He has been an Honorary Lecturer at Queen's University, Belfast for over 20 years, as well as an honorary postgraduate examiner in universities in the UK and overseas. He has held a number of lead training-related roles both locally and for the Royal College of Surgeons of England. He has extensive research experience (with over 50 peer-reviewed publications) and has taught both medical students and postgraduate staff for many years. He has been teaching presentation skills for 20 years.

Julie Terberg is a designer, author, and speaker based in Michigan, USA. She is the founder of Terberg Design, a creative studio focused on crafting presentations. With decades of experience in the industry, she has had trusted partnerships with other presentation professionals and valued clients around the world. Since 2005, she has been recognised as a Microsoft PowerPoint MVP for her contributions to the presentation community.

Echo Swinford began her PowerPoint career in 1997, working for a medical education communications company in the United States. She holds a master's degree in new media from Indiana University and is the owner of Echosvoice, a PowerPoint consulting firm specialising in custom template development, presentation creation, makeovers and cleanup, as well as training for large and small corporate clients. She's been recognised as a Microsoft PowerPoint MVP since 2000 and is President Emerita of the Presentation Guild, a not-for-profit trade association for the presentation industry, which she founded in 2015.

Who is this book for?

Let's be honest. Many doctors, nurses and others involved in healthcare are pretty terrible at presentation design. How could anyone expect otherwise when presentation design is rarely taught?

This book is for all of you, including pharmacists, physiotherapists, dietitians, psychologists, radiographers—we could go on—and yes, even managers. **Especially managers!**

You will have spent years learning how to take a history from a patient, what questions to ask and how to frame them. You will practice how to record these details and how to present them. What is relevant, and what can be left out? It takes a lot of trial and error to get it right, make it engaging and sell your story of the most likely diagnosis or the most relevant investigations.

Now think how much time was spent learning presentation skills and how you put together slides. Is teaching others or presenting your research data any less important? Do you regurgitate a list of facts, or do you tell a story? Do you **sell** your message?

The annual PowerPoint survey developed by Dave Paradi[1] confirms what we have all experienced. Presentations are often boring; they tend to contain a "brain dump" with too many words, typically in full sentences, which the speaker reads off the slides. The text may be too small for the audience to read easily. Visuals, when used, tend to be overly complex. Images are all too often fuzzy, failing to complement the other content or enhance the message. Many visuals are used without recognition that they are subject to copyright.

If any of this chimes with your experience as a presenter, this book is for you. This book will take you through the preparation of a presentation from conception to delivery. You do not need to have any existing expertise with PowerPoint to use this book. Nor does previous experience prevent you from learning more and improving your presentations.

We have included instructions for both Mac and Windows, so don't worry which system you use. Where there are notable differences, we include Mac and Windows screenshots.

The authors are using Microsoft® PowerPoint® for Microsoft 365 (previously Office 365). If you haven't moved to this latest version yet, the screen captures in this book may look a little different than your interface. Don't worry; most of the commands are the same or very similar in earlier versions of PowerPoint. We'll point out any newer features unavailable in older versions. This could be a great time to upgrade.

As we write this book artificial intelligence is beginning to make inroads into presentation design. Microsoft will have released Co-Pilot for PowerPoint by the time you read this. While this is an amazing use of technology, you will still need to design and edit your content to ensure your message is clear. AI will not replace the need for the detailed understanding that this book delivers.

Finally we will introduce you to some of the truly amazing features in Microsoft 365 that will cause your audience to ask how you did that. All we ask is that you tell them about this book.

PART 1

Planning and preparation

Cognitive load and One Big Idea

In a practical book about PowerPoint, starting with a chapter on educational theory may seem odd. Don't be put off if you aren't into educational theory. This is a short chapter with a simple message—"One Big Idea". Cognitive overload is the most common mistake made in presentations, particularly medical presentations.

Studies have shown that if spoken information is presented without visuals, only 10% of it is recalled three days later. If visuals are added, recall increases to 65%.[1] Adding a story to your presentation ensures a further increase in recall.[2]

The message is that a presentation based on dry data alone will not be memorable. It needs visual prompts and/or a story.

ONE BIG IDEA

What do you want your audience to do? This may be to learn more about the subject (you might need a handout, see Chapter 20), to take some action (such as a change in practice), or to give you something you need (more resources probably).

Nancy Duarte introduced the concept of One Big Idea in her book Resonate[3]; this is how we develop a goal for our presentation. The goal should be a single sentence that articulates what you want the audience to do or to take away from your presentation. There are three components to One Big Idea:

1. Articulate your point of view.
   You are a senior figure in health and social care policy, and you need more resources to cope with ever-increasing demand. Your message is not: "I'm going to talk about bed blocking in secondary care". It is: "The failure to support and fund social care is creating a bed-blocking crisis".

DOI: 10.1201/9781003287902-2

2. Convey what is at stake.

This may be a positive thing: "By adopting my suggestions, we can free 80 beds in acute medicine alone", or it may be negative: "If we don't change now, this winter will see ambulances unable to unload outside the Emergency Department".

3. Make it a complete sentence.

By condensing your One Big Idea into a single sentence, you focus your planning for the content. You also give yourself ideas for a crisp finish, but more on that in Chapter 3.

We will return to the One Big Idea concept throughout this book.

COGNITIVE LOAD

Most of you will have eaten in a restaurant chain, where the menu offers choices similar to all the other restaurant chains and where the food is bland and padded out with carbohydrates. Compare that with Spanish tapas, which is traditional "street food". You are served delicious small plates, each different from the others but with a strong culinary theme throughout. The boring, text-heavy, bloated presentation that we all suffer through is the cheap restaurant; the tapas menu is your future slide deck. Each slide has just the right amount of beautifully crafted content, and a constant theme runs through the "meal" to pull it together and give it structure.

Those who are familiar with Sweller's Cognitive Load Theory[4,5] will understand the concept of cognitive overload and the need to consider this in presentation design. Think of cognitive overload as that bloated feeling you have after that unpleasant, cheap meal! Information overload causes the audience's attention to drift or induces somnolence. Breaking your talk into digestible segments makes it more memorable—like good tapas.

Modality

While Cognitive Load Theory suggests that working memory is limited, maximal efficiency is obtained by processing visual and auditory information separately. Indeed, these items are processed in different pathways in the brain. This use of combined images and text is called the Modality Effect.[6] Perhaps this also explains why the combination of wonderful taste and smell, with great-looking dishes, makes tapas memorable (Figure 1.1).

Thus, if visual information (an image, a chart, a diagram, etc.) is provided alongside relevant auditory information (what you say), this is retained better in working memory than the same information in spoken and written format.

This may all be because you are pulling together the function of the left brain (which primarily deals with learning patterns) and the right brain (which is the creative side, dealing with emotion, decision-making, and creativity).

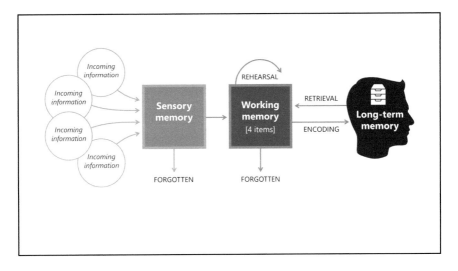

Figure 1.1 Embedding information in long-term memory is a complex process. (Atkinson, R.C. and Shiffrin, R.M. 1968. Image based on a design by Daniel Braithwaite and used with permission.)

Redundancy

Providing the same information in writing on a slide and then reading it out reduces the likelihood of it being retained (Redundancy Effect[7]). That is not to say you should avoid all text on your slides. As you will learn later in this book, a few words in a large, easily readable font can get the message across just as easily as an image, sometimes even better.

To avoid cognitive overload, every element on every slide should have a purpose. Forget that "every slide must have a title" nonsense. If a title isn't needed, delete it. That is one less thing for the audience to read and be distracted by. Replace the title with a call to action or an active title in other circumstances. A few words can let the viewer grasp what the slide is saying instantly.

For example, rather than a standard title saying: "Shift over-runs", try this. Use grey for all the data elements in a chart. Now recolour the group(s) that are over-running their hours in a bold colour (dark red or blue work well). Minimise distraction in the chart by deleting unnecessary elements. Now try adding an active title rather than a generic title (Figure 1.2).

USING EXISTING SCHEMA

For inexperienced learners, in particular, new information that is linked to existing schema is much more efficiently processed in working memory. This emphasises the importance of relating new learning to existing knowledge. All teaching

5

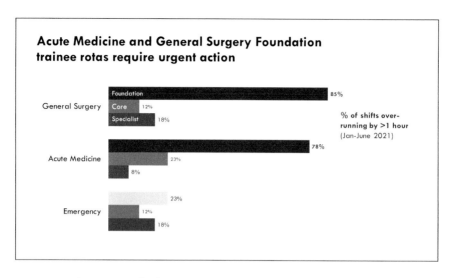

Figure 1.2 Create visuals that viewers can understand at a glance.

should, therefore, start with an understanding of the existing knowledge base of the learners.

For example, you are teaching students about hypertension. It will be much easier for them to understand the causes and treatment if they have already understood the renin-angiotensin mechanism.

HOW DOES THIS WORK IN PRACTICE?

Your talk needs to be sharply focused. You should include only what is absolutely necessary for your audience. To achieve this, you must ruthlessly declutter the content. This means not only removing some of what you say but also all distracting slide elements that contribute to cognitive overload. Resist adding pictures of your children or pets; don't add irrelevant animation.

Let's look at an example. This slide could be used to talk about base-of-skull fracture in a patient on anticoagulation (Figure 1.3).

However, given what we have learned about Cognitive Load, would it not be better to look for an image of "raccoon eyes" and simply present the history, accompanied by an image, perhaps with a take-home message on the slide?

Seeing raccoon (panda) eyes will hopefully help the learner remember the aetiology when they next see a patient with two black eyes. The history does not need to be written down; it is easy to talk it through. After all, that is what we do at the bedside every day.

Case discussion

- A 36 year-old woman is admitted with a depressed level of consciousness.
- She lives alone.
- She has a history of binge drinking.
- Her only past history is of atrial fibrillation.
- She is unsure of her medication.
- Examination is normal with the exception of two rather dramatic black eyes.
- What is the most likely diagnosis?

Figure 1.3 Too much text makes this slide boring.

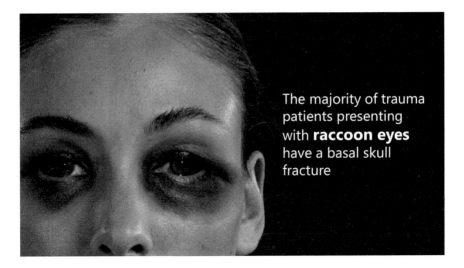

The majority of trauma patients presenting with **raccoon eyes** have a basal skull fracture

Figure 1.4 Keep the text to a minimum and tell the story.

Of course, what is that "One Big Idea"? In this case, it is easy. Racoon eyes in a trauma patient mean there is almost certainly a basal skull fracture (Figure 1.4).

FINALLY

You need to ensure that your message has been understood. In the case of students, you can check this with questions, by asking learners to summarise the key learning, or even with a short quiz.

SUMMARY

The message from this chapter is relatively simple, even if cognitive load theory seems complex! When designing presentations:

1. Understand the existing knowledge base of your learners.
2. Identify their learning needs – The gap in knowledge that you want to fill.
3. If they have learnt one system, try to build on that system (schema) rather than introducing an alternative.
4. Keep your slides simple, clean, image-rich and engaging.
5. Minimise the amount of text on your slides and design them so you can't read them out loud unless the text is short and re-emphasises a key message.
6. Optimise the text size on your slides so that it is legible.
7. Don't put too much information in your presentation.
8. Avoid distractions such as too many colours and animations.
9. Summarise your key points at the end.
10. Emphasise your "One Big Idea".
11. Ask questions to ensure that your message is understood.

NOTES

1. John Medina, Brain Rules, www.brainrules.net
2. Jennifer Aaker, https://youtu.be/9X0weDMh9C4
3. Nancy Duarte, Resonate, Wiley 2010.
4. https://doi.org/10.1207/s15516709cog1202_4
5. https://en.wikipedia.org/wiki/Cognitive_load
6. https://en.wikipedia.org/wiki/Modality_effect
7. https://www.tandfonline.com/doi/abs/10.1207/s1532690xci0804_2

2

Planning your presentation

You may remember with trepidation the first presentation you gave. We're guessing it was awful—ours certainly were! It gets easier with practice, but many healthcare workers develop bad habits along the way. For many, a presentation is just a series of slides to be read out loud. That simply won't do, but how do you avoid this?

In his wonderful book The Presentation of Original Work in Medicine and Biology, published in 1977, Professor Hugh Dudley wrote: "A paper presented verbally will not remain intelligible if it contains as much written communication, or is composed in the same style, as that for publication". Dudley recognised that you must summarise your data and "sell" your key messages, not regurgitate all your research.

As a recently appointed consultant back in 1990, Terry recalls watching the American surgeon John Bascom give a remarkable presentation on the management of pilonidal sepsis. This common condition was regarded as rather trivial, and the surgery was often delegated to inexperienced surgeons. The procedure of choice was to lay open the abscess in the mid-line in the depths of the inter-natal cleft. Healing was always slow and unpleasant; in some cases, young active patients were left with a malodorous, unhealed wound.

In a presentation packed with surgical images and diagrams and very little text, Bascom proposed a radical rethink—incisions should be made away from the mid-line and surgery less radical. His mantra was "Keep out of the ditch", by which he meant the depths of the inter-natal cleft. That was over 30 years ago, and the presentation is still fresh in memory. Why? Because the message was clear and there was One Big Idea—"Keep out of the ditch".

The One Big Idea for this chapter is really easy to remember: Don't open PowerPoint until you have fully planned your presentation. Why not? There are two simple but important reasons: First, if you open PowerPoint, you will be tempted to start typing and write a script for what you will say (and likely end up reading it aloud). The second reason? If you invest time designing a cool slide,

DOI: 10.1201/9781003287902-3

you will be reluctant to discard it, even if it is redundant. We will show you a better way.

PLAN, DON'T TYPE

Normally doctors start putting together a presentation by sitting down at their computer and typing the title of their talk, followed by their name, all onto a white slide. Then they move on to slide two, typing lots of text. This approach makes it difficult to see the overall structure of your presentation. You need to take a step back.

Take yourself somewhere free from distractions—in the park, in the bath, on a comfortable seat or lying in the garden. Ask yourself some fundamental questions about this presentation.

- What are you talking about?
- What does your audience already know about this topic?
- What do you feel they ought to know?
- How much of that knowledge can you reasonably provide in this talk?
- How much time will the presentation take, including questions?
- How much time have you been given (they may not be the same)?
- How important is your talk?
- How will you deliver the talk: At a podium, seated in a small room, or online?

What are you talking about?

Having mulled over these questions, it's time to decide your take-home messages. Think of these as your learning objectives. Can you write them down? Can you summarise your talk with four or fewer key takeaways? More than four can result in cognitive overload, and the audience will remember less of your message.

The learning objectives will drive your takeaway messages, but you should also write down your One Big Idea—your version of "Keep out of the ditch"—to help keep you on track. Be clear about the boundaries that have been set for you. Be ruthless and stick to the task.

How much detail?

Decide what level of detail is required; is this a teaching session for junior medical students, a talk to a patient charity, or a keynote lecture at an international conference? These will obviously be very different.

Table 2.1 Possible headings for teaching about a condition

Theory	Prevention	Diagnosis	Management	Follow-up
Definition	Primary	History	Step by step	Monitoring
Aetiology	Screening	Investigation	Emerging	Complications
Pathophysiology	Lifestyle	Differential	Guidelines	Prognosis
Classification		Approach	Evidence	
		Guidelines		
		Case history		

Table 2.2 Headings for students. You couldn't teach all of these in one go

Theory	Prevention	Diagnosis	Management	Follow-up
Definition	Primary	History	Step by step	Monitoring
Aetiology	Screening	Investigation	Emerging	Complications
Pathophysiology	Lifestyle	Differential	Guidelines	Prognosis
Classification		Approach	Evidence	
		Guidelines		
		Case history		

For example, let's look at a range of broad categories for a medical presentation on a specific disease (Table 2.1).

If you were teaching medical students in their early years, you could not (and hopefully would not) wish to cover all these headings. For example, you might focus on basic theory and diagnosis, to begin with. Here the audience will probably have very little existing knowledge, so keep things simple and short. Remember, avoid cognitive overload (Table 2.2).

If you try to cram all of this into a single talk, you will drown the learners in information, so perhaps talk about some of it and suggest further reading. Or provide some reading before your talk and plan a more interactive style of slide deck to tease out your key learning points.

A common mistake among senior doctors is teaching medical students and trainees far too much about their own specialty because they regard it as important. Is it really that important to a generalist? Indeed, might we put students off our specialty by making it appear too complex?

However, the approach will be very different in giving an update to senior colleagues,, perhaps using these headings instead (Table 2.3).

Table 2.3 **Headings for senior colleagues**

Theory	Prevention	Diagnosis	Management	Follow-up
Definition	Primary	History	Step by step	Monitoring
Aetiology	Screening	Investigation	Emerging	Complications
Pathophysiology	Lifestyle	Differential	Guidelines	Prognosis
Classification		Approach	Evidence	
		Guidelines		
		Case history		

How much time do you have?

Quite frankly, it is rude to overrun your allotted time. This is unacceptable even if you are teaching students or talking to colleagues. The students may have another class to get to and will get in trouble for being late. Your colleagues are busy people. At a conference, the chairman and next speaker will always thank you for finishing early!

How important is your talk?

All presentations are important, but some are more important than others. The time that you take to put the talk together should take into account its importance.

Maybe your talk is for students or your regular induction session. In this case you might reuse it many times. That talk is worth a lot more effort. Spend plenty of time on it and plan it well in advance.

Perhaps you are speaking in a prize session at a major national conference. Or maybe you are applying for a permanent post. You will (probably) only give this talk once, but it means a lot to you; give it the respect it is due.

If this is a talk for the weekly team meeting, you cannot plan it a month in advance—but you can design the slide deck in advance and think about how you will present the data. If you develop a standard layout, the weekly task will be much easier. Indeed, if you develop a layout for this, your slides will look the same every month, so people will "get" your message more easily with time, and you will have your own style available. (See Chapter 14 for how to develop your own unique slide layout.)

How will you deliver your talk?

If you are standing at a podium in front of a large audience, your talk will, of necessity, be didactic. If you are seated in a room with a small group, you can make your presentation interactive.

Do you need to point at slide elements to highlight them? How will you do that—and is it even possible in that environment?

HANDOUTS

Does your talk have to include every detail of your data, or would it be better to have a broad-brush approach? For example, in talking to the hospital board about your latest business plan, you will probably need detailed data. However, when presenting to students, a few key numbers are all you (and they) need, though they will really appreciate a handout.

An accompanying handout is better than cramming all the data into your slides. You could provide this detailed document in advance, then summarise only the most notable data on the slides and refer to the handout to put it in context. Chapter 16 will help you with creative ideas for data visualisation and in Chapter 20 you will learn how to make a great handout.

PLAN A STRUCTURE

Your presentation must have a defined structure. If you are unclear where you are going, the audience certainly won't be able to follow along!

Tradition dictates that for scientific research, this is a title slide, background and/or introduction, materials and methods, results and discussion. Don't confuse these sections. You should not start discussing your results during the methods section or your methodology during the discussion.

When teaching, the convention is to say what you are going to teach, teach it and then summarise what you have taught. In essence, this is about using repetition to ensure that your take-home messages are well embedded.

The rules are more flexible for other presentations, such as audits. However, there is no reason for you to be constrained by any rules if you think you can deliver a more engaging presentation another way.

Kurnoff and Lazarus[1] suggest a structure based on four "signposts". The **setting** represents the background or issue that you are addressing. Then you can introduce the **characters** who participate in your story. This can be you, a named individual or team, a group (e.g. acute physicians or a patient or patient cohort). Next is the **conflict**. What are the issues that must be overcome or addressed? Finally, you should propose a **resolution**.

BUILDING THE PRESENTATION STRUCTURE

At this stage you will need a system to gather your thoughts into the skeleton of a presentation. We will let you open your laptop and start up PowerPoint now, but the reason will surprise you.

Using PowerPoint to plan

Open PowerPoint and insert three blank, unformatted slides. Now print some handouts. These aren't handouts you'd leave behind for the audience. Here we're leveraging PowerPoint's handouts to help us organise and build our presentation.

On a Mac, use the commands **File** > Print (or [⌘] + P), and click on PowerPoint if necessary, to show the dropdown menu. Next, in the Layout section choose Handouts (three slides per page). Set copies to 10 and click Print (Figure 2.1).

On Windows, click **File** > Print (or Ctrl + P) and choose three Slides in the Handouts section of the first menu. Set copies to ten and click Print (Figure 2.2).

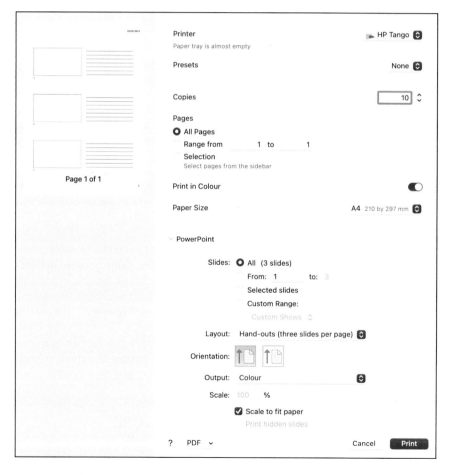

Figure 2.1 **The print menu on Mac.**

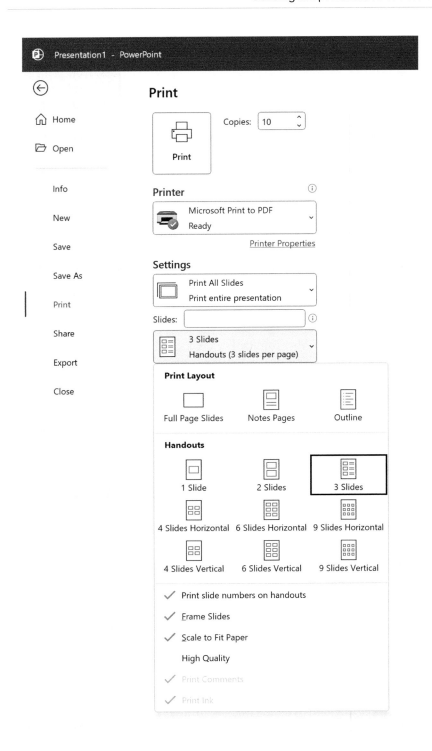

Figure 2.2 The print menu on Windows.

You now have ten pages, each containing three blank slide thumbnails with room for notes beside them.

Now, close PowerPoint. Yes, close PowerPoint. It's best to avoid temptation!

At this stage you can begin to put your presentation down on paper. In the blank thumbnail, scribble a word or two to indicate what will be on the slide. This may be a picture, a chart, a few words or a video. On the lines, write short notes about what you plan to say.

Using Post-It notes to plan

You can achieve the same thing using Post-It™ notes. Scribble what you plan to put on your slide on each Post-It note, rearrange them as you plan and revise your talk.

PUTTING IT INTO PRACTICE

OK, let's look at a practical example. A trainee is preparing a talk on hospital-acquired infections (HAIs). This has been requested because of a recent increase in cases of *C. difficile* infections on the unit. How might this talk be structured?

Clearly there might be a title slide, ideally with visual appeal rather than black text on a white background. Next is an introduction setting out the impact of HAIs, perhaps in terms of mortality, hospital bed occupancy and cost. This will be an overview relating to all HAIs. Here is our **setting**.

It would be impossible to cover every single organism responsible for HAIs, so it is logical to focus on the most relevant ones. If presenting to a surgical group, surgical site infections are important, but for a medical team, not so. However, the on-call medical team might need to know that intra-abdominal sepsis is a potential cause of physiological deterioration, including, for example, atrial fibrillation in the post-operative period.

Our presentation might include data on MRSA, *C. difficile*, hospital-acquired pneumonia, COVID-19 and perhaps Norovirus and Rotavirus. The presentation should have clear section breaks between each of these topics. The design of these section breaks should be similar to tell the audience that the topic is now changing and to break the material into manageable chunks of information. These organisms can represent your **characters**, though you can include patients and staff under this heading as an alternative.

The presenter will need to decide whether to cover all of this or to focus only on *C. difficile*. That will depend on the brief and the time available. Let's assume that the instruction is to cover a range of organisms and then focus on a recent audit relating to *C. difficile*.

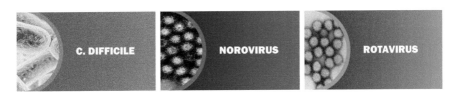

Figure 2.3 Section breaks tell your audience that you have changed "characters".

As the presentation moves between organisms, section breaks will help the audience refocus on the change of topic (Figure 2.3).

What is the **conflict**? Perhaps you are concerned that staff are not following infection control guidelines. Maybe there is a shortage of PPE, or access to handwashing is remote from the patient areas. Are staff returning to work too soon after illness? Is the number of staff on leave creating staff shortages?

As to the **resolution**? We can't help you with that; you need to come up with these solutions yourself!

Here is our outline for this talk

Taking the things we've discussed above into consideration, here is our planned outline for this talk.

- Title slide
- Introduction setting out the magnitude of the problem of HAIs in general and the recent issues in the unit
- Section 1: MRSA
- Section 2: *C. difficile*
- Section 3: Hospital-acquired pneumonia
- Section 4: Norovirus
- Section 5: Rotavirus
- Section 6: Hygiene measures and their impact
- Section 7: Service audit of hygiene measures
- Summary
- Call to action

One Big Idea

Going back to the very beginning, as you outline your presentation, check frequently to ensure that it still focuses on the One Big Idea and supports the key takeaway messages. You want the audience to walk away knowing the answer to the question, "*What was that talk about?*" The response should be your One Big Idea.

Let's assume that our service audit showed that a recent outbreak of *C. difficile* was related to a failure to isolate patients newly admitted to the unit. In this instance our One Big Idea would be as simple as "*We need to be stricter about isolating newly admitted patients with diarrhoea*".

Create a shopping list

Once you have outlined what you are going to say, based on your Post-It notes or thumbnail notes, you can develop a shopping list of items that you need. This may be a laboratory image, some data, a chart from that data or a picture of a patient (with consent). Gather these items in a folder as you prepare to work in PowerPoint.

REHEARSE AND POLISH

You can use your Post-It notes or handout thumbnails and notes to practice your presentation. This will help you to ensure that it flows, to confirm it has a clear structure, and to test the timing. As you do so, you can change your Post-It notes, perhaps altering the order and the content or even delete some things.

You haven't invested time and energy in making a beautiful slide; crumpling up a Post-It note is much easier than omitting a slide that took you hours to put together!

FINALLY, YOU CAN OPEN POWERPOINT!

Only at this stage should you begin building your presentation in PowerPoint. Without a clearly defined structure and careful planning of the order of slides, you may lose focus and leave your audience confused by your message.

The philosopher Pascal[2] recognised the secret to effective communication is not only brevity but carefully focused brevity when he said, "*I would have written a shorter letter, but I did not have time*".

With PowerPoint presentations, take the time. Make it shorter, leaner, and more engaging as a consequence.

NOTES

1. Everyday Business Storytelling. Janine Kurnoff and Lee Lazarus. Wiley 2021.
2. This quotation has been attributed to many others!

3

Starting and finishing with impact

Picture this scenario. You have a presentation to give at an interview, perhaps for a new training post or to secure tenure at a new hospital. The topic set is "**The importance of soft skills in surgery**".

The panel had already interviewed several candidates and is beginning to get a little jaded. You open your laptop, spend a few seconds finding the file for your talk and double-click to open it in PowerPoint.

While your hand is shaking with nerves, you try to position the mouse over the Slide Show icon and click. This all takes 30 seconds, but it feels like 30 minutes[1].

Your first slide comes on screen and looks the same as the last five candidates (Figure 3.1).

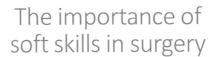

The importance of
soft skills in surgery

Dr. Job Applicant

Figure 3.1 **That boring title slide.**

DOI: 10.1201/9781003287902-4

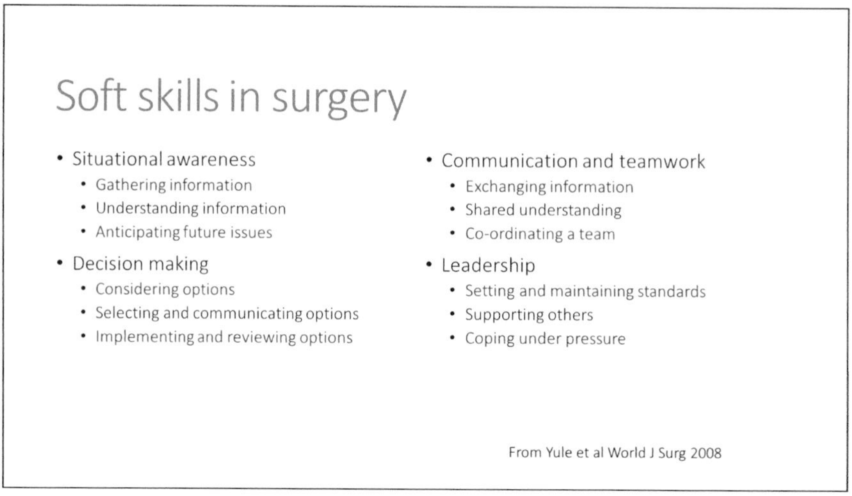

Figure 3.2 **The second slide, based on research by Yule et al.**

You thank the panel, just as the previous candidates have done, read the title out loud, just as they have done, and move to your second slide. This lists some bullet points based on research by Yule et al. This is a busy, text-heavy slide (Figure 3.2).

As you begin to speak, the panel members scan down your text, distracting them from what you are saying. They have seen similar slides from earlier candidates. You are all just going through the motions now.

Is this how you want to start your interview? Will this make you stand out from the rest of the applicants?

So, let's look at the various ways to start a presentation. Then we will revisit this interview and learn how we could do it better.

FIRST IMPRESSIONS LAST

Your presentation doesn't start with your first slide; it begins as you walk in the door or up to the podium. Have you dressed appropriately? This may be "smart casual" or it may require a suit. That is for you to judge.

You should introduce yourself if necessary. What introduction is best? Are you Dr Hannah, or are you Joe, a Core Trainee? Will your relaxed style annoy the older doctors at the front?

Try to smile and project confidence, even if you are screaming inside!

Capture their attention from the very start

You have less than a minute before your audience will decide whether to pay attention to what you are saying, so you can't afford to waste any time.

If you are talking to a small group and the room and topic allow it, talk to them as they arrive; perhaps ask them about today's talk. Try to maintain eye contact. Maybe learn some names so that you can personalise your talk. *"James was telling me that when you saw a patient with jaundice last week, some of you were a little confused about the liver function tests. Let's go over the case and make this easy to understand."*

Clearly at a job interview, this sort of interaction would not be appropriate.

What's next? Most commonly, you'll pull up your first slide.

OPENINGS

So, what makes a great first slide for a presentation? There is no easy answer to this question, but we know it when we see it!

What you put on your slide should be visually appealing and will probably have the title of your talk set against a nice **image**. It is definitely not a white slide with a title and your name in black text!

Options for openings

Traditional medical teaching states that you should start by telling the audience what you are going to tell them. This may be OK, but it is not the only or even the most interesting way to start.

You could begin with a challenge to your audience: *"We are pretty hopeless when it comes to planning long-stay patient discharge."* It might be a call to action: *"I'd like to present a five-point action plan to improve the efficiency of ward rounds."* It may be a wake-up call: *"There have been significant changes in the recommendations for managing peri-operative diabetes. I'm going to summarise these for you today."*

You might consider a quotation to start your presentation. However, beware of overused quotes, and make sure that if you do use one, it is relevant to your topic.

If you are teaching students or trainees on a subject that they often find complex, try something like: *"I'm going to give you a simple guide to help you understand acid-base balance."* It might help if you establish your credentials for this task. In the case of acid-base balance, tell them that you found the teaching on this to be overly complex when you were at their stage. You struggled with it yourself, so you will teach a simple way to understand it.

We often start presentation skills courses with some polling to assess the attendees' existing knowledge and expertise. If you pose some questions to a group of students or trainees, keep the questions simple. Polling is a great icebreaker.

Beware of starting with a joke, this can go horribly wrong. One person's humour is another's offence. It takes an experienced speaker to pull off humour.

Similarly, starting with a shock can work (but it is risky). In general, it may be OK if the shock relates to something external to the group. For example, *"I'm scheduled to talk to you today for 20 minutes about patient safety. According to a study from Johns Hopkins, by the time I have finished speaking, about ten patients in the USA will have died due to medical error."*

A great way to start is with the words *"Imagine if…"* or *"What if…"* You will need to pause after you have posed this question. *"What if we could reduce waiting lists by 20% without spending any money or running any extra clinics?"* We're all anxious to hear more about this!

Give the listeners time to think through their internal responses. Silence is hard when you are speaking, but it's a powerful tool.

Some of the most engaging presentations start with a story if time permits.

Similarly, if you plan to start with some questions, be aware that you may be faced with an awkward silence. This immediately deflates the mood in the room. It is a good idea to warn the audience first; try telling them the question is coming. *"I'm going to start with a few questions to see how much you know already. Don't worry, it's not a test. James, in a minute I want you to tell me what you understand by the term apoptosis."* Give James time to think before you come back to him.

Get to the point promptly

While your first slide sets the scene, the second slide will be the real key to how the talk will go down. You need to make sure that as you move on from your opening statement, the second and subsequent slides keep the audience focussed on you and your message. If your slide is just a word dump, there will be a collective sigh and you will have lost the audience before you even started. We will cover ideas for slide designs that you can use in subsequent chapters.

The bottom line is that the start of your presentation is the hook that catches the audience. You are off to a great start if you can get it right. Conversely, a bad start will likely result in a descent into fidgeting and inattention.

Take note of how other speakers start and learn from them, good or bad.

NOW LET'S REVISIT THAT JOB INTERVIEW

Aristotle argued that persuasion requires three elements: Ethos, pathos and logos. These refer to ethical appeal (establish your credibility), emotional appeal (engage with the audience) and logical appeal (bringing your arguments together in a logical and structured fashion). Can we bring these ideas into our presentation?

As our hypothetical job applicant, you might think of an example of soft skills that you have witnessed. Perhaps you have witnessed things go horribly wrong, resulting in patient harm or even an avoidable death. Maybe you can think of an example that was publicised?

If this was a personal experience of patient harm that you want to use as an example, you could then opt for a full-frame image with bold title text instead of that boring title slide (Figure 3.3).

Your personal story will be more engaging than a list of cold facts. In this case your story is supported by slides that enhance your message and don't distract the panel. At the same time, you're showing that not only do you know the subject, but you have real-world experience. More importantly, you're connecting with the panel and provoking emotion.

As you come to the end of your story you can crystalise your thoughts on this case. These, combined with your personal story, demonstrate your understanding of the issues and how non-technical skills might have prevented patients from being harmed.

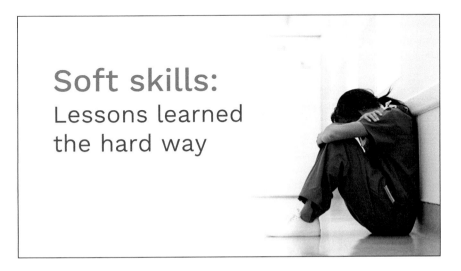

Figure 3.3 A better opening slide.

23

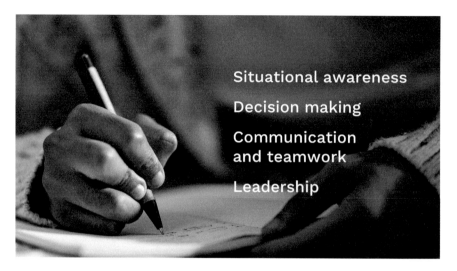

Figure 3.4 Make your second slide easy to understand at a glance.

Now you can show your second slide, which ties your personal experience into the existing science. Here you've used another full-frame image, using the same headings as the poor slide example from the start of this chapter: *"Let's examine this case under four headings as described by Yule"* (Figure 3.4).

You don't need the secondary bullet points you see in Figure 3.2; you know what they are (or can add them to your speaker notes). Keep this second slide clean and simple.

FINISHING

Of course, just because this chapter focusses on the start of your talk, don't lose sight of the fact that the finish is as important as the start.

There are two key messages about your finish. Firstly, make sure that it is clear to your listeners that you have finished. Second, leave your audience with your One Big Idea.

Strange as it sounds, it is often unclear to the audience whether a speaker is done. They stop speaking, but the audience (or chair) doesn't know that this is the end, so there is an awkward silence before anything happens.

This is also an issue for the technical support at meetings. The speaker stops, but have they truly finished? Can the technical support team close the presentation and load the next one? Should they switch on the chairman's microphone? Do they turn the lights up? A simple "Thank you for your attention" may be all you need here.

A clean finish

How might you achieve a clean, crisp finish? Here are a few examples. Note that they are not only a great finish but also contain that One Big Idea:

In closing, I want to leave you with this thought. If we reduced unnecessary prescribing by 20% as I have outlined, we could save enough each month to employ one more nurse per ward.

Thank you for listening to me. I hope that I have also encouraged you to listen to and learn from complaints. Complaints are how we improve our service, not a distraction from patient care.

Or perhaps just a warning that you are about to finish:

I'm going to finish with a short quotation from Homer (the Greek, not the Simpson); I hope you will remember this the next time you see a confused elderly patient. *Our value lies in what we are and what we have been, not in our ability to recite the recent past.*

TAKING QUESTIONS

If you are taking questions from the audience, you might want to repeat the question before you answer—even if there's a roaming mic. Not only will this clue in others who may have missed the question, but repeating or rephrasing it ensures that you have heard and understood the question before you begin answering it.

Be sure to wrap up the questions in time to repeat your One Big Idea and close your presentation cleanly.

SUMMARY

Hopefully this chapter has given you a clearer understanding of the importance of the start and finish of your presentation. Those few minutes at the start are the hook that catches the audience's attention and draws them in. The last few minutes are the stamp that embeds your message.

NOTES

1. In Chapter 18 we will show you a much better way to start up your presentation.

4

Where to find images

Images make or break a presentation. In this chapter we will help you find the images that will enrich your presentation. In Chapter 7 you will learn how best to use them.

WHAT ARE THE DIFFERENT IMAGE TYPES?

Most readers will not be familiar with the common file formats for images, so it is worth explaining these briefly.

Raster images

These images have a defined resolution (size to you and me). If you enlarge the image so that it is stretched above this resolution, it will start to pixelate and look fuzzy. We have all seen this many times in presentations. Common types of raster images include the following:

JPEG *(Joint Photographic Expert Group)*: You may see this as a file extension .jpeg or .jpg – they are both JPEGs. This is probably the most common file type used in PowerPoint. As a rule, you will need a JPEG with a horizontal dimension of about 2000 pixels to fill a slide at high quality. You can scale this down so a 1000-pixel wide image could look good across half the slide, and so on.

PNG *(Portable Network Graphics)*: The advantage of PNG files is the ability to support transparency (Figure 4.1). However, the same concerns apply regarding resolution, so you will still want at least 2000 pixels across the image to fill the slide.

GIF *(Graphics Interchange Format)*: OK, first off, it's pronounced JIF with a soft G! GIFs are familiar to most social media users as they are often animated. You can create GIFs in PowerPoint, but it takes a bit of effort. They are less useful when inserted in PowerPoint for several reasons. GIFs are limited to 256 colours and the appearance and animation can seem rather amateur. You can't create transparency or crop them. Animated GIFs play automatically, so you can't use timings as you can with video. Finally, they are usually awful!

DOI: 10.1201/9781003287902-5

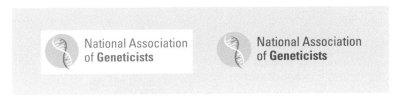

Figure 4.1 A JPEG usually has a white box around the logo, as JPEGs do not support transparency.

TIFF *(Tagged Image File Format):* TIFF files are uncompressed image files. They are rarely seen in PowerPoint, as they can be very large files.

BMP: Bitmap images are composed of dots (like images in an old newspaper). They are rarely used now because of their poor quality.

Vector images

These images are made up of mathematically derived shapes to describe their content. The beauty of vector images (often called SVG or scalable vector graphics) is that they can be resized without losing resolution. A good example of a vector image is an icon inserted from the PowerPoint icons menu.

SVG images can also be converted to shapes, and this is particularly useful with diagrams. For example, this image of the anatomy of the heart is available from Wikimedia (Image Wapcaplet, Yaddah – Own work, CC BY-SA 3.0, https://commons.wikimedia.org/w/index.php?curid=830246) (Figure 4.2).

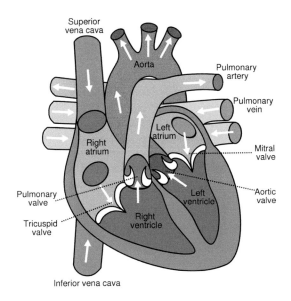

Figure 4.2 A PNG image from Wikimedia.

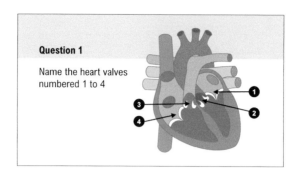

Figure 4.3 Our modified slide with the labels removed.

You cannot easily remove the labels from this image as it is a PNG. You can, however, download the image as an SVG from Wikimedia and insert that onto your slide instead. Then right-click the SVG and choose Convert to Shape. Now each element of the shape can be altered, moved, or deleted. We were able to remove the text labels and make the slide in Figure 4.3 in just a few seconds.

EPS: Encapsulated Postscript. This vector file format is designed to work across software programmes, particularly the Adobe design suite. It produces high-quality images suitable for presentations or print. They cannot be inserted directly into PowerPoint.

EMF and WMF: Enhanced Metafile and Windows Metafile. These legacy vector formats can be inserted into PowerPoint on Windows, but they don't work on Mac. SVG is a much better file format to use these days!

PDF: Portable Document Format. PDF is the older method of inserting vector images into PowerPoint on Mac. SVG has replaced this in modern versions of PowerPoint. Because PDF allows documents to be viewed on virtually any platform without any design software, it can be very useful when you're distributing PowerPoint files.

Icons: Icons are easily added from the PowerPoint Insert ribbon, though the range of medical icons is currently somewhat limited. We would recommend The Noun Project for a greater range of icons. If you are a student or educator, they will offer you an educational discount on your subscription. There is also a PowerPoint add-in for The Noun Project. (https://thenounproject.com).

A great source of free medical-style icons is the Health Icons website (www.healthicons.org). The range of icons is again rather limited, but if you have a specific need, you can request additional icons through the site.

Further sources of free icons include Flat Icon (https://flaticon.com), Google icons (https://fonts.google.com/icons), Remix (https://remixicon.com), and Reshot (www.reshot.com).

When you use icons, remember that less is more—you don't need an icon for everything! Also, try to choose icons that have the same style characteristics. This will make your presentation look more professional.

CHOOSING THE RIGHT IMAGE

What makes a good image? That is a tough question.

Design is very subjective, but we can certainly give some thoughts on the types of images you will find useful and those that just won't work. Fussy, busy images are generally unsuitable for use in PowerPoint, even if they are great images (Figure 4.4).

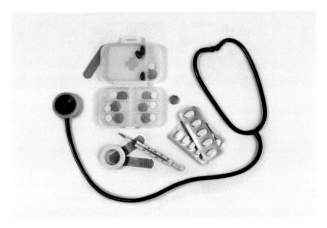

Figure 4.4 A nice image, but not great for use in PowerPoint. This image from Julie Zyablova from Unsplash is wonderful, but there is just too much going on to use it in a presentation.

What message does this image convey? Where would we place the text?

On the other hand, Figure 4.5 from JD Mason, also on Unsplash, is ideal. There is a beautiful dark background, with lots of room to place our message. This area is called white space (even though it is not white). White space gives your slide content room to breathe, resulting in a more impactful message.

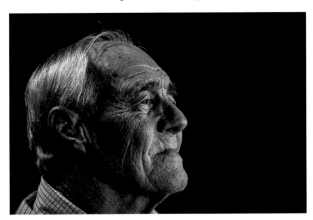

Figure 4.5 This image has lots of "white space". Image from JD Mason on Unsplash.

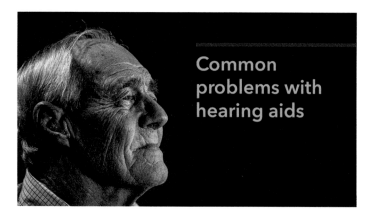

Figure 4.6 The image used as a title slide or section divider.

It is easy to envision a title slide using this picture (Figure 4.6).

Beware of images that might irritate the viewer. A quick search on Unsplash will reveal lots of images of syringes. However, many show vaccines in 10ml syringes (ouch!) or with air still in the syringe (oops!). Many stock sites contain cliched images. Some surgical scenes appear to show surgical staff in unsterile nitrile gloves. So be careful in your image selection.

It is worth mentioning here that your choice of images also needs to be cognisant of gender, racial, sexual, age and other stereotyping that comes under the heading of unconscious bias.

HIGH-QUALITY PHOTOGRAPHIC IMAGES

You may be familiar with the term royalty-free stock photography. We generally use royalty-free images in presentations, which just means you pay once to use the image. The important thing to understand is that royalty-free doesn't necessarily mean cost-free.

That said, many sites offer a wide range of royalty-free images both for *free* and for *fee*. When deciding which images to use in your presentation, it's important to be aware of these differences, respect the owner's copyright, and pay for usage rights as required. Misusing copyrighted images can result in lawsuits, which will definitely cost you more in the long run!

Free stock images

Many websites offer royalty-free stock images for your use at no cost. Usually, you are requested either to acknowledge the author on the slide or share a thank you on social media.

Some of these include Unsplash (www.unsplash.com), Pexels (www.pexels.com) Pixabay (www.pixabay.com), Morguefile (www.morguefile.com), Rawpixel (www.rawpixel.com). Most of these images are not specific to medical-related subjects, but you can still find some useful photos and illustrations.

FREE STOCK IMAGES FROM WITHIN POWERPOINT

You can access stock images from within PowerPoint and use them in your presentations without the need for special licensing or permissions. To insert one of these images, select the **Insert** tab, then click the down arrow beside Picture and select Stock Images. A dialogue box will open, into which you can type your search term. Select your preferred image and choose Insert.

You can also search for Creative Commons images from within PowerPoint by selecting Online Pictures when you use Insert Pictures. Although you can filter to Creative Commons images here, you still need to check the licensing level to ensure that you can use these images with impunity. Read on to learn more about Creative Commons licenses!

CAN I GET MEDICAL IMAGES FOR FREE?

At present there are a few sites that offer royalty-free, cost-free medical images. You will still need to request permission to use some images, so read the terms and conditions carefully.

The Health Education Assets Library (HEAL) is a collection of over 22,000 freely available digital materials for health sciences education (https://library.med. utah.edu/heal/). These include excellent images curated from other collections.

For those with an interest at cellular level, there is Cell Image Library (http:// www.cellimagelibrary.org/home).

Ed Uthman curates an impressive Flickr catalogue of pathology images, and it is a pity he doesn't have a shorter URL! We have made him one: https://tinyurl. com/Ed-Uthman!

The National Library of Medicine runs Open-I (https://openi.nlm.nih.gov) and MedPix (https://medpix.nlm.nih.gov).

It is also worth exploring the Visible Human Project (https://www.nlm.nih.gov/ research/visible/visible_human.html).

The National Cancer Institute has a fantastic range of images at Visuals Online with labels in English or Spanish (https://visualsonline.cancer.gov).

For ophthalmologists, there is the National Eye Institute media library (https:// medialibrary.nei.nih.gov).

The CDC (Centers for Disease Control and Prevention) has a range of images very specific to their role (https://phil.cdc.gov).

Medical images for purchase

Some sites offer medical images for sale, and if your presentation is important, you might want to explore some of these.

A UK site, Shout (https://www.shoutpictures.com/index), charges for images, but they are of very high quality, and you may find exactly what you need if you are involved in emergency medicine.

Medical Images offers a wide range of photos and illustrations (https://www.medicalimages.com), though the price may put you off.

Standard stock image sites

You can also pay for images from standard image stock sites, some of which are listed below:

- iStock Photos   https://www.istockphoto.com
- Getty Images   https://www.gettyimages.com
- Shutterstock (PPT add-in available)   https://www.shutterstock.com
- Adobe Stock (PPT add-in available)   https://stock.adobe.com
- Stocksy   https://www.stocksy.com
- Alamy   https://www.alamy.com
- Cavan Images   https://www.cavanimages.com
- Masterfile   https://www.masterfile.com
- Media Bakery   https://www.mediabakery.com
- Offset (by Shutterstock)   https://www.offset.com
- Superstock   https://www.superstock.com

GOOGLE IMAGES

Many PowerPoint users will head straight for Google and do an image search, but there are caveats to this. Frankly, there are much better sources of images, as we've listed above.

Most images resulting from a Google Image search are copyright-protected and you must not use them for commercial purposes. The definition of "commercial purposes" is unclear. If, for example, you are an invited speaker at a conference and your expenses are paid, that could be construed as commercial purposes. You can probably use images from Google Images under the Fair Use terms for single-use teaching of students, but are you being paid to teach? Is that a commercial use? It's a very grey area.

Creative Commons licensing

Generally, if you're using Google to search for images you can legally use, look for images distributed under a Creative Commons license. Creative Commons licenses allow people to make their works available to the public under a variety of licensing levels. For example, CC0 licensing allows you to use the image as-is or even with modification and requires no attribution to the creator. Other CC license levels may be limited to non-commercial use, disallow modification, or may require attribution to the creator. Generally, you should look for CC0 or Public Domain images, but you can—and should!—read about the different Creative Commons license types at https://creativecommons.org/about/cclicenses/.

Openverse (https://wordpress.org/openverse/) and Wikimedia Commons (https://commons.wikimedia.org) are both useful sites to search for images free to use under Creative Commons licensing. You can also filter your Google Images search using Tools > Usage Rights > Creative Commons licenses to limit your results. Bing Image search offers similar tools; click Filter > License. Be sure to check the license details for your selected image to ensure you understand and comply with the CC attribution requirements. And be careful not to grab an image for purchase because those are often mixed in with the free Creative Commons results! (Read more about that below.)

Image sizes

Often you will find that when you add an image to PowerPoint, it is smaller than your slide and it pixelates when you enlarge it. This is because you have chosen a low-resolution image. You can filter these out in the Google Images search Tools menu. Selecting Size > Large will return somewhat larger, and therefore usually higher-resolution, images.

Advanced search

However, you can be more specific in your search. Search for an image term, for example, "doctor". Now click on the gear icon (for settings) at the top right of the Google page. Click on "Advanced search" and choose an appropriate image size.

In this example we have searched for images of a doctor larger than 1024 pixels by 768 pixels. We've also added options to search for images with a "wide" orientation and have a Creative Commons licence so that we are free to use them without copyright issues (Figure 4.7). Ideally, to ensure a 2000 pixel-wide image, search for images larger than 2 Mbytes.

As we mentioned earlier, you might think this will return only images that you can use for free, but that isn't always the case. Double-check every image you use to ensure it is safe to do so.

Find images with...		To do this in the search box.
all these words:	doctor	Type the important words: winter hoarfrost
this exact word or phrase:		Put exact words in quotes: "frost flower"
any of these words:		Type OR between all the words you want trees OR weeds OR grasses
none of these words:		Put a minus sign just before words that you don't want: -windows

Then narrow your results by...						
image size:	Larger than 1024×768				▼	Find images in any size you need.
aspect ratio:	Wide				▼	Specify the shape of images.
colours in the image:	● any colour	full colour	black & white	transparent	this colour:■	Find images in your preferred colours.
type of image:	any type				▼	Limit the kind of images that you find.
region:	any region				▼	Find images published in a particular region.
site or domain:						Search one site (like sfmoma.org) or limit your results to a domain like .edu, .org or .gov
SafeSearch:	Show explicit results				▼	Tell SafeSearch whether to filter sexually explicit content.
file type:	any format				▼	Find images in the format that you prefer.
usage rights:	Creative Commons licences				▼	Find images that you are free to use.

Advanced Search

Figure 4.7 Google Image search.

Reverse image searching

Because free and for-purchase images are often combined in image search results, it may be a good idea to err on the safe side and check the heritage of an image by reverse image searching using Google Lens (https://www.google.com/imghp?hl=en&ogbl). Again, Bing and other search engines also have similar reverse image search tools (Figure 4.8).

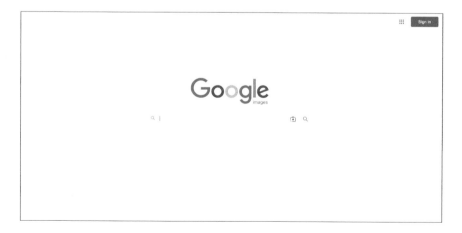

Figure 4.8 Click the camera icon to do a reverse image search.

Please do not put images in your slides that have a watermark copyright sign in them! The bottom line is we do not recommend using images from Google image searches.

IMAGES FROM YOUR WORK

Oftentimes you'll have access to images from your work environment that may be accessible and permissible to use. Just be sure to check local guidelines and policies on using these images.

Images of patients and staff members

For images of patients and staff members, it is essential that you obtain signed consent from everyone in the image, not just for the image to be taken but also in respect of every use you plan for the image.

Under no circumstances can you ever take an image of an unconscious patient without written consent. This cannot be sought retrospectively—so just don't do it!

This is a complex legal area, so please don't take these images yourself. Hospitals and other medical facilities will have rules for taking photographs, and you should check the rules for your institution before you take any images. In any case, the medical photography department will probably take much better images for you.

Furthermore, images taken of patients are part of the patients' medical records and must be stored in an unaltered format so that they can be accessed in the future. Do not keep these images on your home computer or phone, and never send clinical images by text or email without written consent from the patient (and only if hospital policy allows this).

There are also technical considerations in taking medical images. For example, before and after comparison images of faces require careful lighting and head positioning. The bottom line is to leave these images to the experts.

Images of equipment

You can use images of medical equipment, but if you download these, be sure that there is no copyright watermark, and look at the website to see if there are any usage restrictions. We find that if you email the equipment or device manufacturer, they are normally more than happy to supply high-resolution images for you to use.

Radiology images

The days of photographing X-ray plates have hopefully long gone. Most hospitals now use PACS. These usually have a facility to export images as JPEG files, which should have the patient details removed from them. In our experience, you simply right-click on an image in the viewer and choose "Save as". Check out your local system; if you are uncertain how to do this, ask a radiologist.

If you must use a radiology image that is not anonymised, be wary of placing a simple black box over the patient identifier. This can easily be accidentally displaced or deliberately removed. Remember, you have a legal and ethical responsibility to avoid breaches of confidentiality.

A better way to anonymise radiology images is to "embed" your black box into the image. Add and position the black rectangle to cover any pertinent information, then select both the radiology image and the black box (hold down shift while clicking on each in turn). Now press (Ctrl [⌘] + X) to cut both objects and add them to the clipboard.

Next, click the arrow next to (Mac) or below (Windows) the **Paste** button on the **Home** tab and select Paste Special. Choose PNG or JPEG. This merges the picture and black box into a single image, which prevents the box from being inadvertently moved or deleted.

Images from surgery or endoscopy

Images that are taken at surgery or endoscopy and in which the patient cannot be identified are generally safe for use in presentations. However, obtaining written consent from the patient for their use is a wise precaution.

Be very careful about using these images. A distinctive tattoo on the patient's skin may be enough to identify them to others.

TAKE YOUR OWN PICTURES

You may be a photographer and can take your own images; indeed, images from modern smartphones are fine for use in PowerPoint. Even if you don't consider yourself a great photographer, there are plenty of opportunities to get suitable images outside of your work environment. For example, the photo used in the slide shown in Figure 4.9 was shot on an iPhone 11.

AI IMAGES

Artificial intelligence is a rapidly expanding area in computing. At the time of writing, AI-generated images vary greatly in quality and accuracy. However,

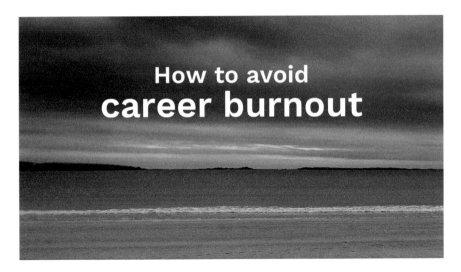

Figure 4.9 An iPhone shot can make a good image for a slide. (Author's own image.)

the technology and tools are progressing at a fast pace, and soon you should be able to prompt AI to generate high-quality images for your presentations. Clear, specific instructions (prompting) are the key to producing the best results. You should carefully examine AI-generated images for technical accuracy and be sure to attribute the AI tool used.

CARTOONS

There are plenty of cartoons available on the Internet. There is no reason why you can't use them in your talk, but, as always, be aware of the potential copyright issues. You should also be conscious that what one person finds amusing might be offensive to another.

You can, of course, commission cartoons from artists if you have a specific idea in mind.

INFOGRAPHICS

Infographics are graphic visual representations of information, data, or knowledge intended to present information quickly and clearly. They can be simple and visually appealing, but when done badly, they can result in complex slides that cause cognitive overload.

There are websites where you can create your own infographics very easily, or you can create them directly in PowerPoint. If you need a complex infographic, it may be worth hiring a graphic designer or a presentation designer to help you develop it.

SUMMARY

Using images is key to effective presentation design, but they must be appropriate for your subject, relevant to what you are discussing when you show the image, and of high enough quality to look professional.

Beware of potential copyright infringement as you search for your images; neglecting this can prove very costly.

Don't be put off despite these caveats. Great images will transform your slides.

PART 2

Constructing your presentation

An introduction to the PowerPoint interface

If you are a novice, you might find the PowerPoint user interface daunting. Don't be afraid to play around with the features. You can't break anything, and it's much safer to practice on a presentation when you have some free time rather than waiting until the day before a major deadline. In our experience, even relatively experienced users can benefit from a more detailed understanding of the learning in this chapter.

HOW WE DISPLAY KEYSTROKES AND COMMANDS

Before we get started, we want to acknowledge that, even though they are very similar, there are still differences between PowerPoint on Mac and Windows systems.

Probably the biggest difference in Microsoft 365 is the existence of an actual menu in Mac PowerPoint, but almost all the tools are also available on the ribbon. Of course, on Windows, the tools are *only* available on the ribbon!

Because the ribbon tools are common between Mac and Windows, we'll use them for most of our instructions. If you're used to using the menu commands on Mac, of course, you can still use them! But if you see, for example, **Insert** > Pictures > Stock Images, then that means to click the **Insert** tab, then the Pictures button, and then the Picture From File option. We have bolded the word **Insert** to show that we are talking about a **tab** on the ribbon.

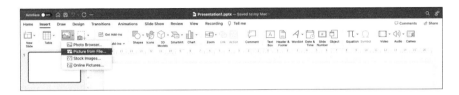

Figure 5.1 A sequence of clicks, **Insert** > Picture > Picture from File.

DOI: 10.1201/9781003287902-7

Sometimes there may be small wording differences in the labels, but it should still be easy for you to understand the sequence on either platform.

In Windows, many shortcuts require that you hold down the Control key **and at the same time** click another key, for example, Z (this is the very useful shortcut for undo). We would use Ctrl + Z to indicate this. On a Mac the same combination uses the Command key, which we'd indicate using ⌘ + Z. Throughout the book, we've used the notation Ctrl [⌘] + Z to cover both options (Figure 5.1).

TABS AND RIBBONS

The critical functions in PowerPoint are accessed from the ribbon. The ribbon appears as a row of labels, which are called tabs.

As you click on a tab, the ribbon will change to reveal commands specific to that tab. For example, the **Insert tab** is (as the name suggests) for inserting things, such as pictures, shapes, icons, charts, or videos. In Figure 5.2, the **Insert** tab is active, and you can see the various tools. The orange line is under the active tab.

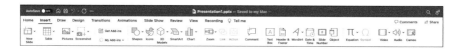

Figure 5.2 **The Insert tab of the ribbon.**

Some tools are duplicated on several tabs of the ribbon. For example, you can perform common tasks such as inserting shapes on the **Home** tab as well.

The ribbon tabs are context-sensitive. If you select text, the **Home** tab will open, as that is where you will most often modify text. If you click on a picture to select it, the **Picture Format tab** will appear. This tab is not visible by default, only when you are modifying a picture. Similarly, the **Video Format** and **Playback** tabs will appear if you select a video (Figure 5.3).

If the tab you want is not visible, you may not have selected the object you wish to edit. Just click on the object and the relevant tab will open. If the tab is visible but not active, you can simply click on the tab to activate it and see the available tools.

If you are a Mac user, there are a series of fixed menu choices above the tabs:

File | Edit | View | Insert | Format | Arrange | Tools | Slide show | Window | Help

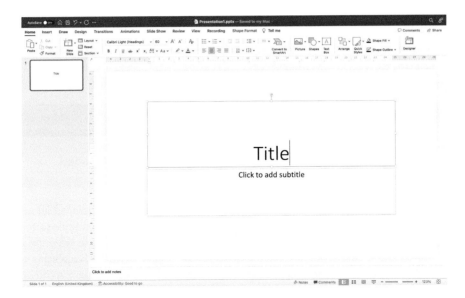

Figure 5.3 The Home tab of the ribbon. Because the cursor is in a placeholder, a context-sensitive tab for Shape Format is also visible, though not currently active.

Since almost all the options in these menus are also available in the tabs, they may seem redundant. However, the File menu is mostly equivalent to the File tab in Windows, so you will need this menu option for some commands that are not found in the tabs (Figure 5.4).

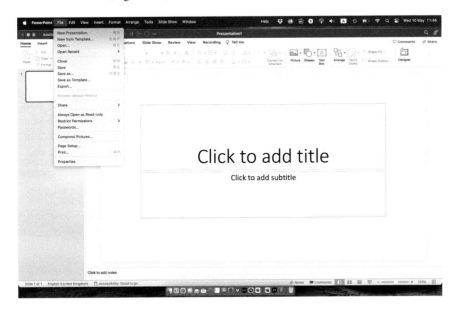

Figure 5.4 The File menu on a Mac is the only way to access several items.

QUICK ACCESS TOOLBAR

In our experience, most presenters are unaware of one of PowerPoint's most valuable features. This is the Quick Access Toolbar or QAT (Figure 5.5).

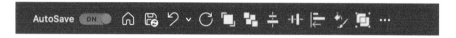

Figure 5.5 The Quick Access Toolbar with additional commands added.

The QAT is the thin toolbar above the ribbon on a Mac. (It can be placed above or below the ribbon in Windows.) You can add your commonly used tools to the QAT. This is particularly useful for commands that require multiple selections. For example, if you frequently use the distribution tools to evenly space objects—see Chapter 9 for this technique in detail—you'd have to click **Home** > Arrange > Align > Distribute Horizontally every time. You can do this with one click of a button on the QAT!

To add tools to the QAT on a Mac, click the ellipsis (three dots) and choose one of the options listed, or choose More Commands to access all the possible tools. On Windows, you can right-click any tool on the ribbon and choose Add to Quick Access Toolbar, or you can right-click in the QAT and choose Customize to access all the possible tools or rearrange the ones you already added. We recommend being selective about which tools you add. The QAT allows one line of tools, so pick the tools that are most useful to you.

We like to add the alignment and distribution tools to our QATs because, as we just explained, they take a lot of clicks to get to. The same goes for the Selection Pane—it's sometimes buried deep in the tools and is much easier to get to from the QAT. We also like to add the Shapes gallery because it's in so many different places on the different ribbon tabs that it's difficult to develop muscle memory for it; putting it on the QAT means it's always there in the same place.

One tip is to add tools to the end of the QAT if you're working on certain types of projects. For example, if you needed to crop a bunch of pictures into squares or circles, you could add the Crop aspect ratio 1:1 and the Crop to Shape tools to your QAT and then remove them when you're finished with that project.

OPENING PowerPoint

You may not realise that you can change the initial view to turn off the Start screen when you open PowerPoint, which bypasses the various stock template options and opens a new blank PowerPoint file directly in Normal view. The Start screen is enabled by default.

To turn it off, on Mac, click the word PowerPoint on the top-level menu, then go to Preferences > General and untick the box for "Open Presentation Gallery when opening PowerPoint". On Windows, untick the box next to **File** > Options > Show the Start screen when this application starts.

Backstage view

If you leave the Start screen enabled, PowerPoint will open to what's known as Backstage, where you find various template, save, and file management options. If you've bypassed the Start screen, you can access these features on Mac by clicking the File menu, and **File** > New from Template will open Backstage itself. On Windows, click the File tab to access.

Normal view

Normal View in PowerPoint is what we think of as the editing view. This is the preferred option for many people on opening PowerPoint because it starts with a blank slide ready to add content.

To your left of the active slide, there will be thumbnails showing a miniature of each of your slides. Dragging the vertical divider between these thumbnails and the active slide area enlarges the thumbnails and reduces the size of the active slide area, or vice versa (Figure 5.6).

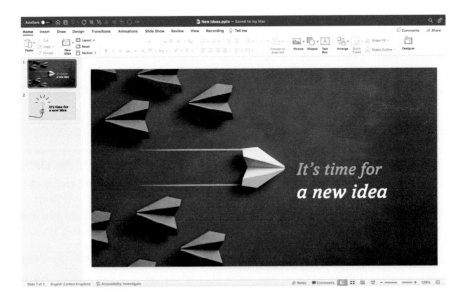

Figure 5.6 **Normal view.**

At the bottom of the window is what's called the status bar. Starting from the left you see the current slide number, and in Mac PowerPoint, the default language. Set this to your own preferred language (including versions of English) by clicking on it, choosing your language, and then selecting "Set as default". In Windows PowerPoint, these settings are on the Review tab. The Accessibility checker is to the right of language.

Towards the right you will see the word "Notes". Here you can toggle between showing or hiding your speaker notes. You can also drag the horizontal divider to increase the size of the notes section. The text you type here will appear in Presenter View.

On the Mac, you can activate the Comments pane from the status bar; on Windows, do this on the Review tab. Comments are used if you are collaborating in constructing a presentation. Next is an icon that toggles between Normal and Outline View—which we rarely use. To the right of this, another icon allows you to toggle between Normal and Slide Sorter View. This can be very useful for reordering your slides. The next icon opens Reading View, which displays the slide show in a window instead of full screen. We sometimes use this during the design process to preview animations.

Most users will be familiar with the icon which opens Slide Show View. Alternatively, you can use the shortcut F5[1] (⌘ + Return) to begin your presentation. If you are in the midst of a slide deck and want to open the current slide in slide show mode, use Shift + F5; on a Mac ⌘ + Return will always open the active slide.

A small slider to the right of the slideshow button can be used to zoom in or out on your active slide area. Alternatively, on a Mac, use ⌘ and + to zoom in and ⌘ and – to zoom out. On Windows, press Ctrl while scrolling your mouse wheel. Zooming in can be helpful in checking accurate alignment (see Chapter 9). To reset the slide area to "Fit to Window", click the right-most icon.

STARTING A NEW PRESENTATION

When you start PowerPoint, the default presentation template is the Office theme. This comprises a white slide background with black text. The font is currently Aptos Display for headings and Aptos for body text. Older versions of PowerPoint may still use Calibri. Sticking to this template and using only text or the default tables and charts is commonplace but results in a boring, generic slide deck.

You can open the **Design** tab and select one of the built-in templates. This is certainly a more appealing look for your slides. However, there are many more templates available to you (Figure 5.7).

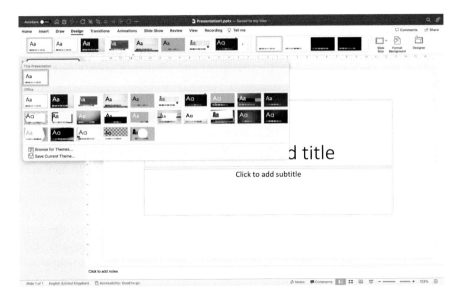

Figure 5.7 The Design tab, showing the built-in templates.

You can search for new templates from Backstage View. Figure 5.8 shows a template found using the search term "Medical" with dummy content.

Once you have downloaded a template, save it on your computer using **File** > Save As Template. Now you can use this template by selecting it from the gallery in Backstage View.

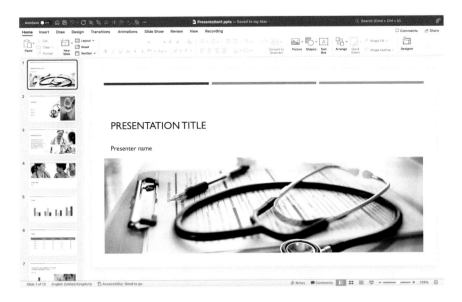

Figure 5.8 A template downloaded from the Microsoft 365 web page.

What are placeholders and layouts?

When you open PowerPoint, you will see that for each slide layout, there are default placeholders. These will usually tell you what they are for. For example, the title layout has text that says, "Click to add title" and "Click to add subtitle".

Do not move these placeholders; otherwise, your slide content will jump about when you advance from one slide to the next. Don't worry if you accidentally nudge or move them; you can use the reset button to get them back to their default position.

The position and look of each placeholder will depend on the slide layout that you have chosen. You select slide layouts from the **Home** tab. If you select the down arrow beside New Slide (or below it on Windows), you can choose from any of the layout options available in the current template. We will cover slide templates in more detail in Chapter 14 (Figure 5.9).

If you want to change the layout of the current slide, you can select Layout, and the layout options will be shown. Click another layout thumbnail to apply it.

Some layouts will give you a placeholder with multiple options for content. The most commonly used is a Title and Content layout, which allows you to select from bullet points, a table, a chart, a SmartArt graphic, a 3D model, a picture from a file on your computer, an online picture, a video from your computer or

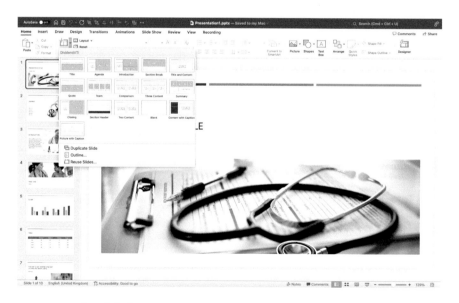

Figure 5.9 The Slide layout gallery using the down arrow beside New Slide.

a stock icon. You can only select one of these. The content you choose will be positioned within the placeholder. Provided you don't move the placeholder, all your slides will have these objects in the same position on the slide, which looks much better. However, this layout tends to encourage you to add bullet point text and isn't always the best choice.

If you plan to add objects to your slides free hand—perhaps in the form of a process diagram or other graphic—it is wise to use the Title Only layout. This will ensure that all your titles are in an identical position on your slides.

The first placeholder you will use will be on your title slide, which includes the instruction "Click to add title". The text that you add will, by default, use the "Headings" font set up in that template. This font is also the default for all titles in subsequent slides.

The remaining fonts throughout your presentation, whether in bulleted text, text boxes, charts or tables, will be the default body text for the chosen template.

We will cover fonts in much more detail in Chapter 13.

SAVING YOUR PRESENTATION

You should save your changes regularly during preparation of any presentation. Even though PowerPoint will attempt to recover your unsaved file, there is nothing worse than having your computer crash after you have modified fifty slides only to find that you failed to save the presentation and you have lost all that work.

You can save your presentation using the keyboard shortcut Ctrl [⌘] + S. This becomes second nature after a while. When saving a file for the first time, you will be shown a dialogue box prompting you to choose a name for your presentation and a place to store it on your computer or online. The name will default to "Presentation1". You do not need to delete this; just type over it. Then carefully select where on your computer you wish to store the file. You may want to create a new folder for any practice files from this book.

You can also use **File** > Save to save and manage your files if you want to change the file name or where it is saved. On PowerPoint for Windows, click the **File** tab; on PowerPoint for Mac, click the File menu to access the various Save options.

We will deal with saving your presentation in a lot more detail in Chapter 12, but we make no apology for duplicating this advice. There is nothing worse than spending time on a presentation and then losing all your hard work.

NOTE

1. Some PCs require Function-F5 to open the slide show

6

Adding shapes, lines, and text

If you are an experienced PowerPoint user, you are probably familiar with using shapes and lines. Even so, there will be a few gems for you in this chapter (some of which we think will change your life!), so stick with us.

Although we will emphasise throughout this book that an image is worth a thousand words, some slides require text, often contained within a shape such as a circle or a rectangle.

A WORD ABOUT PLACEHOLDERS

The default PowerPoint file—as well as almost every template you'll encounter—has built-in placeholders for text and other content. These are the pre-positioned, pre-formatted holders.

You are almost certainly familiar with how to add text to these placeholders. Just click on the text prompt; for example, on a title slide, "Click to add title" and start typing a title.

In a bullet point slide, click where it says "Click to add text" and type away. You can choose to use the default bullet point or select the bullet point gallery on the **Home** tab and choose none if you don't want bullet points.

These placeholders are ideal for bulleted text slides and for charts or diagrams that need to fill the area indicated by the placeholder. However, it can be frustrating when your content doesn't match the placeholder configuration on the slide.

In those situations, click the arrow next to the New Slide button (Mac) or click the bottom of the New Slide button (Windows) on the **Home** tab and see if any of the other layouts with different placeholder configurations will work better for your content. If not, then you may want to opt for a layout with only the title placeholder (usually called Title Only, as you might expect!) so you can add your own shapes and diagrams in the empty areas of the slide.

The reason we recommend that you use the title placeholders to house your slide title text is this helps keep the slide titles from jumping around and distracting

DOI: 10.1201/9781003287902-8

your audience as you move from slide to slide. If you need to adjust the formatting or position of the title (or other) placeholders, see Chapter 14 for an overview of how to customise your template.

ADDING A SHAPE

You can add shapes, lines, and text from the shapes gallery. The easiest way to access this is from the **Home** tab, though you can also access the same options using the **Insert** tab and even many of the contextual tabs. In fact, because the shapes gallery appears in so many different places, it's difficult to develop muscle memory for it. We've added it to our Quick Access Toolbars, so we always know where to find it! Check the information in Chapter 5 for a reminder on how to set up your QAT.

If you click **Insert** > Shapes, you can select your chosen shape in the shapes gallery, then click and drag on the slide to create the shape. You can resize the shape by typing into the input boxes in the size area of the Shape Format tab, or you can drag any of the handles to resize and reshape the shape.

If you want to constrain the aspect ratio of the shape while you resize it, press and hold the Shift key while you drag a corner. On a Mac, you can even tick the Lock Aspect Ratio box on the ribbon to make your life easier!

In Windows, this feature is hidden in **Format Shape** Task Pane > Shape Options > Size > Lock Aspect Ratio, so it's probably easiest to just remember to press Shift while resizing (Figure 6.1).

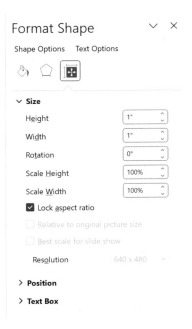

Figure 6.1 To constrain the proportions of a Shape when resizing in Windows, check the box for Lock aspect ratio on the Format Shape task pane.

BUT WHAT IF I WANT A PERFECT CIRCLE?

You may have noticed that there isn't a circle or square shape in the shapes gallery, only ovals and rectangles. That's because a circle is simply an oval with equal height and width, just as a square is a rectangle with equal height and width. To create a perfect square or circle, select the oval or rectangle shape in the gallery and then click anywhere on your slide. PowerPoint will insert a 1 inch (or 2.54 cm) shape—a perfect circle or square. Alternatively, press and hold Shift while you click and drag to create the shape.

Once drawn, use the techniques listed above to maintain the aspect ratio while resizing the shape as needed.

INSERTING LINES

Inserting a line is similar to inserting any other shape. Select one of the line styles in the Shapes Gallery. You have several options, including straight or curved lines, elbow connectors and arrows. Try inserting some of these to see how they work. To be honest, we rarely use anything other than the plain old line. (We don't even use arrows too much; instead, we apply arrowheads to lines using the shape outline options. Read more about those below.)

It can be quite fiddly to keep a line perfectly horizontal or vertical when drawing freehand. Once again, the shift key comes to the rescue! Hold down the shift key before you click on the slide to begin drawing the line. This constrains the line to horizontal, vertical, or 45 degrees in any direction. If you need to vary the line length after it's drawn, just hold the shift key as you do so to maintain the set angle.

CONNECTING SHAPES WITH LINES

Often you will want to draw a series of shapes and connect them using lines. If you simply draw the lines and shapes, they will become disconnected when you move any of the elements on the slide. But you can connect them, so this doesn't happen.

To see how this works, draw two rectangles on your slide. Position one on either side of the slide. From the shapes gallery, select a straight line. When you move your mouse over the slide to begin drawing the line, the cursor will change to crosshairs. Note that as you move the cursor over the shapes on the slide, small dots appear on the shapes. These are your connection points (Figure 6.2).

Click on or near a connection dot on the first rectangle, then drag to a connection dot on the second rectangle. You'll feel the line "latch on" to the shape, and you can test that it's connected by dragging the shape elsewhere on the slide. If the

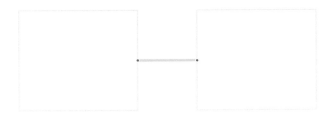

Figure 6.2 When a line is connected to a shape, small dots will appear at the united points.

line moves with it, they're connected. If you're using connected lines, it's important that the connected shapes are perfectly aligned, otherwise, your lines won't be straight. You'll learn about alignment in Chapter 9.

FORMATTING FILLS AND OUTLINES

These will vary depending on the template, but PowerPoint generally applies a default colour fill and line to your shapes. You can change these by selecting the shape, line, or text box and using the tools on the **Shape Format** tab. If one of the pre-set formats in the Shape Styles gallery meets your needs, by all means, click it to apply! Otherwise, you can use the various Shape Fill and Shape Outline options to format your shapes.

Most of the options are pretty obvious, but if you don't find what you want, you can choose "More Options" at the bottom of any of these menus. For example, to apply a 2-pt weight to your shape outline, choose Shape Outline > Weight. Looking at the flyout menu, you'll see there isn't a 2-pt entry. In that case, choose More Lines at the bottom of the flyout to open the Format Pane, and in the pane, go to Shape Options > Fill & Line (the paint bucket icon) > Line, where you can choose from all the possibilities. You can also right-click and choose Format <whatever object> to open the Format Pane, and on Mac systems, there's a Format Pane button on the **Shape Format** tab of the Ribbon that will open it (Figure 6.3).

Basically, PowerPoint makes a bunch of common options available to you from various tabs of the Ribbon, but *all* the formatting options are available in the Format Pane. The nice thing is that these same options can be applied to a variety of content—charts, tables, SmartArt graphics (which are really just a collection of shapes), pictures, icons, you name it!

ADDING SHAPE EFFECTS

Shape effects include embellishments like shadows, reflections and glows. Like the various fill and line settings, shape effects can be accessed from many of the tabs, and they can be applied to multiple types of content. You'll also be able to get to all of the shape effects options in the Format Pane.

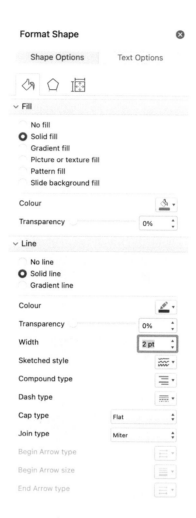

Figure 6.3 The Format pane includes all Formatting options in one location.

As far as we're concerned, shadows are the only shape effects you should use. We know adding decoration is tempting, but the most effective designs are simple; as with everything else, less is more.

USING THE FORMAT PAINTER

Once you've formatted a shape to your liking, you can use the Format Painter tool to apply that formatting to other objects in the file. The Format Painter will change your life! Select your formatted object and click on the paintbrush icon on the **Home** tab to activate the Format Painter. Then click another object on the slide to apply it. Voila! Instant formatting.

Double-click the Format Painter icon to retain the formatting information so you can apply it to multiple objects throughout the presentation. Click ESC when you're ready to disable it.

You can also add Shift to your copy-paste shortcuts to pick up and apply formatting: ⌘ + Shift + C (Mac) and Ctrl + Shift + C (Windows) copy the formatting; ⌘ + Shift + V (Mac) and Ctrl + Shift + V (Windows) apply it.

INSERTING AND FORMATTING TEXT

You can type text into the standard placeholders in the PowerPoint templates, but this doesn't always give us the desired results. So, we often use shapes for text. In fact, you may not realise it, but you can add text to any shape (except for lines). Simply select the shape and start typing.

We like to add text directly to the shapes because doing so generally makes things easier. If we're animating, there's only one object to worry about. If we're rearranging things, there's only one object to worry about. If we're still adding lines and drawing objects, there are fewer shapes to fuss with.

Of course, sometimes it's difficult to get the text positioned exactly where you want it, especially with circles and triangles. In those situations, adding the text in a separate text box can be easier.

To insert a text box onto a slide, click Text Box in the shapes gallery and click and drag on the slide—just as you would for any other shape. Then type your text. Note that PowerPoint does not add any fill colour or outline to text boxes by default.

You can format the text as you would in any other Office programme by selecting the text and choosing your preferred font, font size, colour and text alignment. And you can, of course, add fills and lines to the text boxes in the same way you can add them to shapes.

THE BASICS OF FORMATTING TEXT

Regardless of whether you're working with text in a placeholder, a non-placeholder text box, or a shape, you can apply the same types of formatting features.

Bullets

Placeholder text usually starts with a bullet; non-placeholder text usually doesn't.

You probably already know that you can turn the bullets on and off using the Bullets button on the **Home** tab. Please stick with PowerPoint's simple circles and squares—anything else is just a distraction (Figure 6.4)!

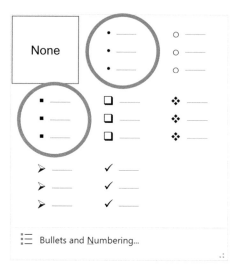

Figure 6.4 When using bullet characters, it's best to choose a simple circle or square.

Creating second-level text is easy if you're working in a placeholder. Because placeholders are designed to hold multiple levels of text, you can simply press Tab at the beginning of the line before you start typing, and the text will pick up the second-level text formatting and spacing from the template. Note that this doesn't work if your first-level text doesn't have a bullet character. In that case, click the Increase Indent button on the **Home** tab to create second-level text.

Text boxes you add from the Shapes Gallery are not designed to hold multiple levels of text, so all indents and formatting will be manually performed. Use the Increase Indent button or the indent carets to create second-level text and then apply the formatting you need.

Notice that we're not discussing anything below second-level text? That's because anything lower than the second level should be considered a talking point and not included on your slides! And, the truth is, a lot of times, you should move even the second-level text from the slide into your talking points.

Fixing hanging indents

Sometimes when you add or remove bullets, the hanging indents get messed up. These are easy to fix, especially once you head to the **View** tab and turn on your ruler!

Use the carets on the ruler to control your text indents. Drag the top of the upward-pointing arrow to add or decrease the space between the bullet and the text (Figure 6.5).

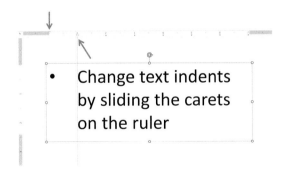

Figure 6.5 **Adjust text indents by sliding the carets on the ruler.**

Line spacing

In PowerPoint, line spacing refers to how close together the lines of text are. You can see what settings are used in **Home** > Line Spacing > Line Spacing Options. For maximum readability, stick with Single or Multiple .9 here.

Spacing Before and Spacing After refers to the space between bullet points or paragraphs of text. Increasing this can help the user distinguish between text entries and sometimes eliminate the need for a bullet point altogether.

You don't have to use both before and after spacing. Choose one and go with it! A good rule of thumb is to use anywhere between 6 to 24 pt space before, depending on the size of the text. For example, if your text is 20 pt, 12 to 18 pt spacing usually looks good. This is, of course, only necessary if you have more than one "paragraph" of text in your text box or placeholder (Figure 6.6).

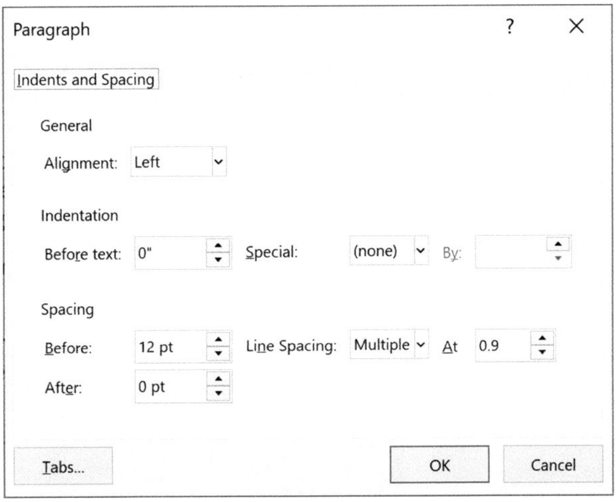

Figure 6.6 **Adjustments to line and paragraph spacing can help make your text easier to read.**

Do not autofit

Sometimes when you try to resize a shape or a text box, it won't stick and instead snaps back to whatever size it started at. This is completely annoying! You can fix it by selecting the option to "Do not Autofit," which can be found in the Format Pane under Text Options > Text Box or Shape Options > Size & Properties > Text Box.

By the way, *shrink text on overflow* is the setting that's responsible when you type too much text into a placeholder, shape, or text box, and it becomes extremely small and the line spacing becomes super tight. You can also fix that by selecting *do not autofit* instead and then resizing the text manually or, better still, deleting some of your text.

Horizontal (paragraph) alignment

Stick with left-aligned text; you'll never go wrong. Because we read left-to-right, left-aligned text is the easiest for us to read. Occasionally we'll use centred headings, but only with small bits of text. The same goes for all capital letters; reserve this for small bits of text.

Although PowerPoint lets you right-align and justify your text, we don't recommend using them, as they can both be difficult to read and don't usually enhance your design.

VERTICAL ALIGNMENT AND MARGINS

When you're positioning text, whether it's included directly in a shape or in its own text box, you may need to change the vertical alignment. This will determine whether the text is anchored at the top, the bottom, or the middle of the text box or shape. To adjust this, select from the Align Text options near the horizontal text alignment buttons on the **Home** tab (Figure 6.7).

Margins are the blank space or padding inside a shape that keeps text away from the edges. Once you start working with text and shapes, you may realise that adjusting the margins can often help you position things more easily.

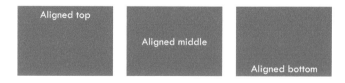

Figure 6.7 Text can be aligned vertically to the top, middle, or bottom of a text box or shape.

Unfortunately, the internal text margin settings are buried: Find them in the Format Pane under Text Options > Text Box or Shape Options > Size & Properties > Text Box. We often set the margins of text boxes to 0 on all sides to make them easier to align with each other and other shapes on the slide. Note however, that text within a shape needs a little room around the edges to allow it to breathe (Figure 6.8).

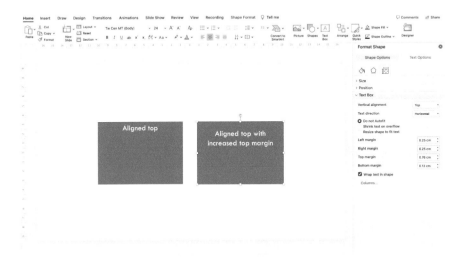

Figure 6.8 Adjusting the internal margins on shapes can help better position text within them.

LAYERING OBJECTS

When you add objects to your slide, PowerPoint layers them, with the newest objects at the top. So, if you create a shape and then a text box, you can easily drag the text box on top of the shape. But if you created the text box first, it will be behind the shape. We call this ordering of objects the Z-order (Figure 6.9).

You can see the objects all listed in order on the Selection Pane, which you can enable on the **Home** tab, the **Shape Format** tab, or any other tab where you find the various Arrange tools. If you select an object in the pane, it will be selected on the slide and vice-versa. This can help you identify specific objects in a sea of similarly named bits! In fact you can also click to select an object in the pane and then click again to select the text and rename it. This is especially helpful if you're animating because those new names appear in the animation pane as well.

Hiding shapes by clicking the eyeball icon can help you select shapes hiding behind other shapes. Clicking the lock button is handy for temporarily preventing you from selecting objects and inadvertently moving them as you're working.

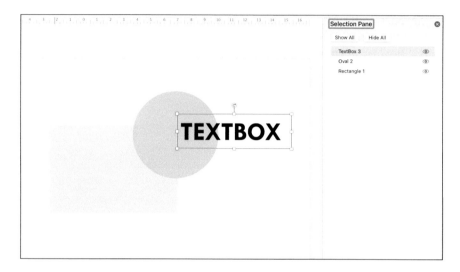

Figure 6.9 The selection pane displays a list of all objects on the slide in a front-to-back order.

You can move objects behind other objects in a number of different ways: Select and drag them in the selection pane, use the up and down arrows in the selection pane or use the Send to Back/Bring to Front buttons in the Arrange tools. Send Backward and Bring Forward move the objects layer by layer, while Send to Back and Bring to Front move things all the way to the bottom or top layer at once. You can see these in action if you open the Selection Pane and check the order of the objects as you use the various tools.

Mac PowerPoint also has a nifty Reorder Objects tool on the Shape Format tab that shows your slide in 3D layers, which can really help you visualise how the various objects relate to one another and then adjust their Z-order.

SmartArt AS STARTER ART

SmartArt graphics can be useful for displaying text in something other than just a basic bulleted list. But they can also be pretty clunky and fiddly to format.

We often use SmartArt as a starting point to turn a bulleted list of text into shapes that we can easily format.

Try this: Take one of your existing slides with lots of text in bullet points or insert a new slide, choosing the Title and Content layout. Type some text into the body placeholder. Now right-click in the text and hover over Convert to SmartArt (Windows only) or use **Home** > Convert to SmartArt. Choose an appropriate diagram. For this text, the Horizontal Bullet List is a good starting point (Figure 6.10).

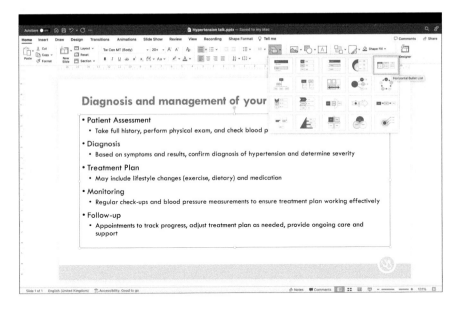

Figure 6.10 SmartArt can be a good idea-starter to change a basic bulleted list into a better visual.

At first glance, this SmartArt graphic doesn't look too bad. But if you put on your designer hat, you can see that this could be improved. Here we used **SmartArt Design** > Change Colours to select one of the "colourful" options (Figure 6.11).

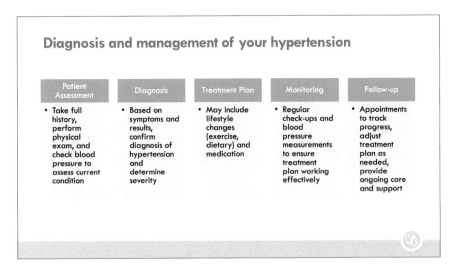

Figure 6.11 The bulleted text converted to a SmartArt graphic.

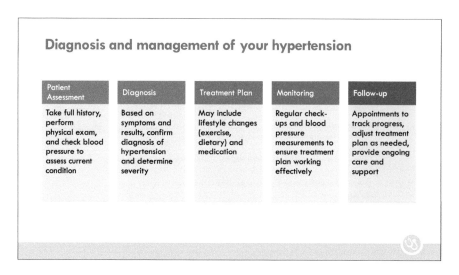

Figure 6.12 Using a SmartArt graphic as a starting point, you can apply some simple formatting changes for better results.

Make a few simple tweaks, such as bolding and left-aligning the headings and removing the unnecessary bullet characters. Please resist choosing a SmartArt style from the gallery, as most of those effects are overdone and dated. If you need to make extensive changes, select the SmartArt and on the **SmartArt** tab, choose Convert > Convert to shapes to make things easier to format and arrange (Figure 6.12).

7

Inserting and editing images and icons

Getting rid of text-heavy slides is the key to an engaging presentation; the solution is often to use an appropriate image or icon.

WHY USE IMAGES

There is no doubt that adding images to your presentation makes it look prettier, but that is not the main reason to do so. You may recall from Chapter 1 that learners remember more if you combine text with images. This enables them to embed knowledge more easily. Using images also stops the audience from reading text-heavy slides and lets them focus on you, the presenter.

Let's look at this slide defining learning disability, used with permission of the original author (Figure 7.1).

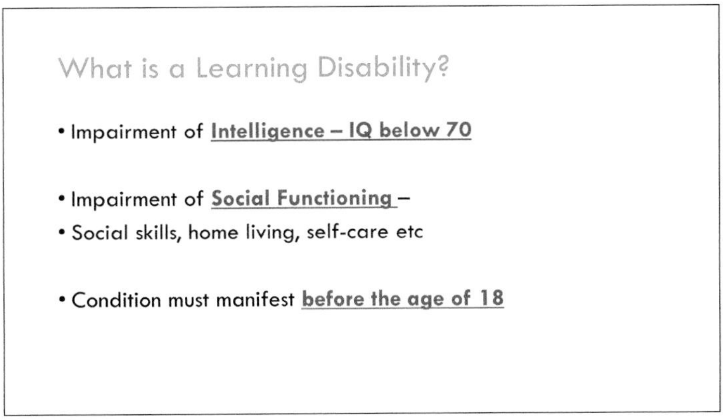

What is a Learning Disability?

• Impairment of **Intelligence – IQ below 70**

• Impairment of **Social Functioning –**
• Social skills, home living, self-care etc

• Condition must manifest **before the age of 18**

Figure 7.1 A standard bullet point slide.

DOI: 10.1201/9781003287902-9

It covers the definition of learning disability but doesn't set the world alight. If we think about the content, the three statements in red are the key messages. The presenter has underlined them and used a red font to emphasise them, but what they are illustrating is that the black text is redundant. Wouldn't it be better to put those few relevant words over a meaningful image (Figure 7.2)?

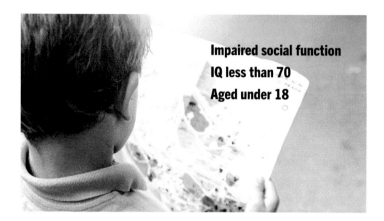

Figure 7.2 Using an image with limited text results in a much more engaging slide.

INSERTING IMAGES ON YOUR COMPUTER

You may have images saved on your computer. Just be sure that they are safe for you to use and that you are not infringing copyright.

Images of your own: You may have an image that has been saved from your PACS service or taken by the Medical Photographer.

Images you have downloaded: As described in Chapter 4, you can search for an image of high enough resolution to fill your slide and download it to your computer. Be sure to save it somewhere that will enable you to find it again.

Inserting these images is very simple. Go to the **Insert** tab and choose Picture > From File. Navigate to the image file, highlight it and click Insert.

INSERTING POWERPOINT STOCK IMAGES

We covered this in Chapter 4, but here's a quick reminder. In the **Insert** tab, choose Pictures > Stock Images and use the search box to look for a suitable image. These images are of high enough resolution to fill your slide without pixelation.

MY IMAGE DOESN'T FIT THE SLIDE

When you add an image, it rarely fills the slide by default.

Images that are too small for the slide

If the image is very small and you stretch it to fill the screen, you may distort it, so be sure to hold the shift key down as you enlarge it (on a Mac, tick the Lock Aspect Ratio box next to the image dimensions on the Picture Format tab) (Figure 7.3).

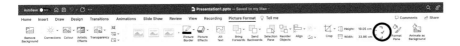

Figure 7.3 The Picture Format tab and the tick box that locks the aspect ratio on a Mac (to the right of the height and width).

However, dragging a small image to fill the slide commonly results in pixelation (fuzziness) of the image. This is because the number of pixels in the image is too small. You cannot fix this; the best solution is to look for a higher-resolution image (Figure 7.4).

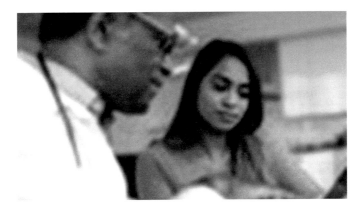

Figure 7.4 A pixelated image where image resolution is too low.

Images that have the wrong aspect ratio

Commonly the image is not the same aspect ratio as your slide. To fill a widescreen slide, we usually use an aspect ratio of 16:9. However, most images have a different aspect ratio. You will need to crop it rather than distorting the image to fit (Figure 7.5).

CROP TO ASPECT RATIO

We downloaded the rock-climbing image from the PowerPoint stock images. However, it doesn't match the widescreen format. To fix this, select the image and from the **Picture Format** tab, click the arrow beside "Crop" and choose Aspect Ratio > 16:9. Click anywhere outside the picture to accept the changes. After cropping, you

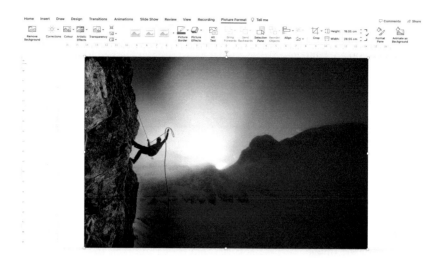

Figure 7.5 This picture inserted from Microsoft Stock Images doesn't quite fill the slide area.

can resize the picture to fill the slide. Select the picture and move it to the top left corner of the slide. Then press and hold Shift while you drag the lower right corner of the picture to resize, meeting the bottom right corner of the slide (Figure 7.6).

CROPPING TO OTHER SIZES

Of course, you may not need the image to fill the slide. In that case you can crop to whatever dimension you require. The freehand crop tool will suffice. Simply click Crop and then drag the crop marks to achieve the best result for your needs.

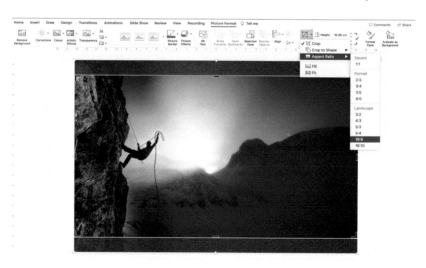

Figure 7.6 Here you can see the setup to crop a picture to a 16:9 aspect ratio, which is the same as the default PowerPoint slide.

You can also drag the picture within the crop marks to reposition the subject. Or click and drag the white corner handles on the picture itself to resize it within the crop frame. Once you are happy, click outside the image to accept the crop (Figure 7.7).

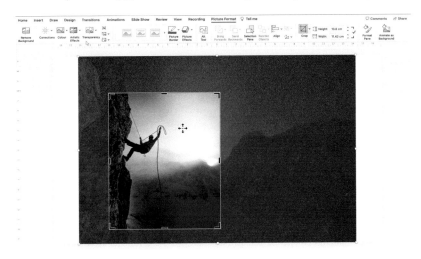

Figure 7.7 You can use the crop tools to edit the picture size and to reposition the picture within the new cropped area.

CROPPING TO OTHER SHAPES

You don't need to crop the image to a rectangle. You can choose to crop to any shape you wish using the Crop To Shape option. Just bear in mind that if you want to crop to a perfect circle, you need to crop to an aspect ratio of 1:1 and then crop to an oval (because a circle is an oval with a 1:1 aspect ratio) (Figure 7.8).

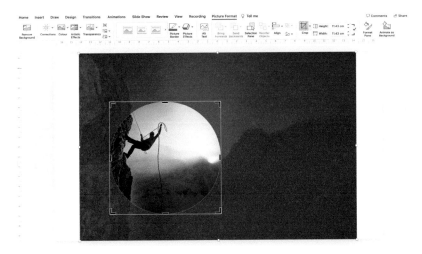

Figure 7.8 Crop to a perfect circle by cropping to an aspect ratio of 1:1, then Crop to Shape and select Oval.

ADDING WHITE SPACE TO AN IMAGE

On occasion you will find an image that is great for adding text, but there is not quite enough white space for the text. White space, you will recall, is the uncluttered area of an image—it does not need to be white.

Crop and stretch part of the background

If a picture doesn't quite fill the slide and you don't want to crop out any part of the subject, you can try using a portion of the picture to fill in the gap. This technique won't work with all images, but it's sometimes handy for adding white space.

In Figure 7.9, you can see that the picture of the doctor doesn't quite fill the slide. We could crop the image to 16:9 to fill the slide, but that would crop out too much of our subject and won't have enough room on either side for text.

Working with a copy of the image perfectly aligned with the original underneath it, crop to an uncluttered part of the background, as you see in Figure 7.9. Keep the newly cropped image in the same position, grab the sizing handle on the centre-left and stretch the slice to fill the open area of the slide (Figure 7.10). (This is the one and only time it's okay to stretch an image!)

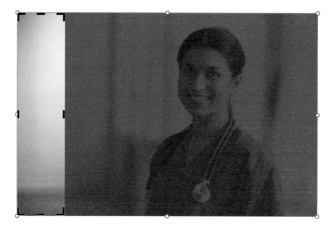

Figure 7.9 Using a copy of the picture, crop a slice on one side of the image.

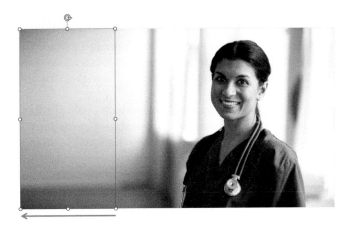

Figure 7.10 Stretch a copy of the background image to fill the rest of the slide, creating white space for text.

Crop and enlarge part of the image for the background

Another technique to create white space is to use part of the image for the background. The mountain climbing picture features a dark blue area on the lower right. Working with a copy of the original picture, resize the image within the 16:9 crop frame to include only the dark blue area. Click away to accept the crop, then enlarge this background image to fill the slide. Even though this background area might not be as crisp when it's enlarged, that's okay—background images can be a little blurry, and this provides us with more uncluttered space to include supporting text (Figure 7.11).

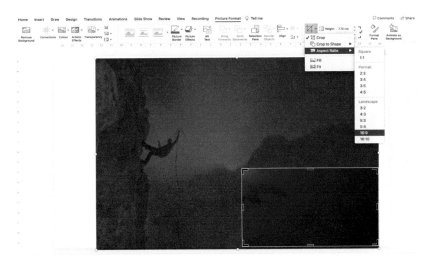

Figure 7.11 Crop an uncluttered portion of the picture and resize it to fill the slide, creating white space for text. Note that the crop is to an aspect ratio that will fill the slide area when enlarged, in this case, 16:9.

OTHER EDITING CONSIDERATIONS

Once your image is on your slide, the tools you used to modify any shape are the same tools that you can use on your image. You can add an outline and/or shadow. You can alter the colour and thickness of the outline (Figure 7.12).

Additionally, PowerPoint supplies you with various tools to edit pictures. The correction tools have options to lighten, darken, sharpen and soften images, and the colour tools have pre-sets to alter saturation and tone or to recolour images (Figure 7.13).

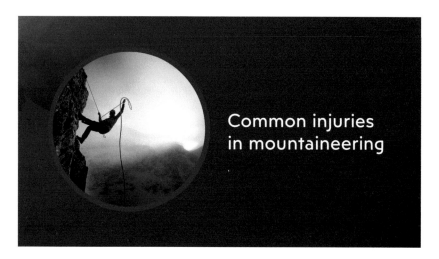

Figure 7.12 The picture has been cropped to a circle, has had an outline added, and has been placed on the left to provide white space for text.

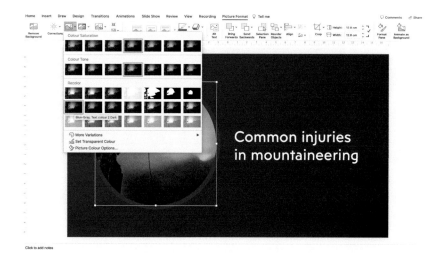

Figure 7.13 The colour options in the Colour Gallery.

REDUCING FILE SIZE

Be aware that digital images can be huge. Including more than a few pictures can bloat your presentation and make it impossible to email or place a strain on older processors when you are editing or presenting.

You may need to compress the images in your presentation to reduce file size. To do this, go to **File** > Compress Pictures. You then need to consider which options to choose.

If you are showing your presentation on a very high-resolution screen, you may wish to retain High Fidelity or select HD 330 PPI as the picture quality setting. But for most purposes, Print or On Screen will suffice and result in smaller files. Deleting cropped areas of pictures will also reduce file size, but it cannot be undone later. Do you have a backup of the images in case you regret this?

You may choose to compress all the pictures in your presentation rather than only the currently selected picture. Be sure to double-check the file after compressing to ensure your photos still look good.

NXPower Lite

Alternatively, consider purchasing a programme to compress your presentation. We strongly commend NXPower Lite. This software will compress any Microsoft Office file and produce a copy so that your original is preserved, allowing you to go back and recover those cropped images if you need to. Note: For files less than 50 MB, you can use their free online compressor at wecompress.com

ICONS

A common challenge for medical presentations is finding an image that matches your message. Sometimes it's impossible, and in that situation, icons come to the rescue.

Let's use some icons in a practical example. We all see slides like Figure 7.14 every day.

What are the key messages? We've highlighted them in Figure 7.15. It's difficult to make slides visual when there's too much text, so the plan is to keep the key messages on the slide and move everything else to the speaker notes area.

Scanning text in smaller chunks is much easier, so we've developed a slide with a coloured, full-frame background image and added text boxes with our key messages (Figure 7.16).

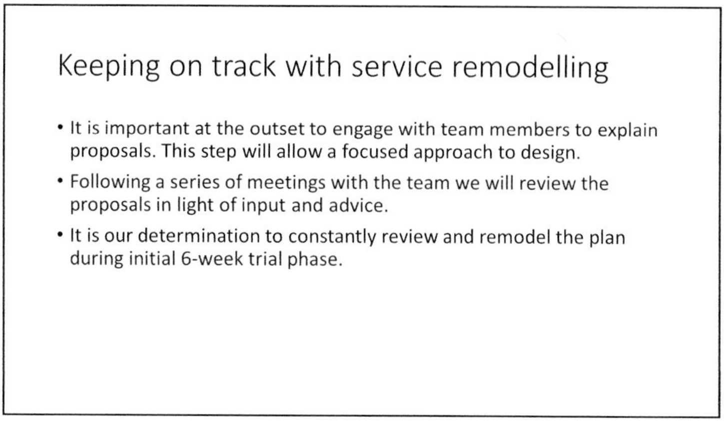

Keeping on track with service remodelling
• It is important at the outset to engage with team members to explain proposals. This step will allow a focused approach to design.
• Following a series of meetings with the team we will review the proposals in light of input and advice.
• It is our determination to constantly review and remodel the plan during initial 6-week trial phase.

Figure 7.14 Another boring bullet point slide.

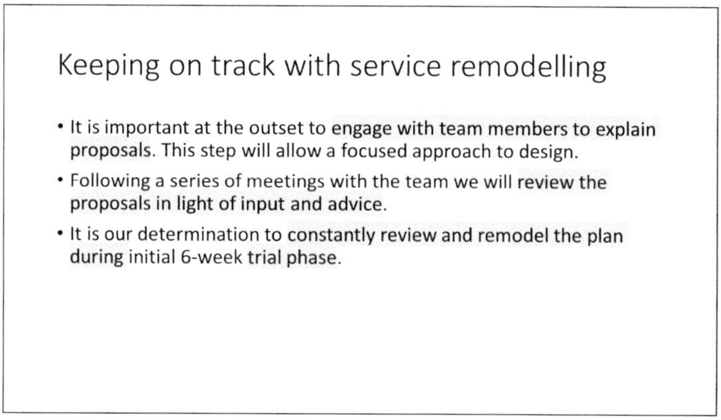

Keeping on track with service remodelling
• It is important at the outset to engage with team members to explain proposals. This step will allow a focused approach to design.
• Following a series of meetings with the team we will review the proposals in light of input and advice.
• It is our determination to constantly review and remodel the plan during initial 6-week trial phase.

Figure 7.15 Key messages highlighted.

Keeping on track with service remodelling
Engage with team members to explain proposals
Review proposals in light of team input and advice
Constantly review and remodel during trial phase

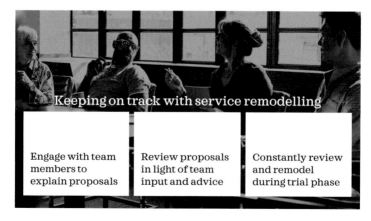

Figure 7.16 The key messages transferred to text boxes.

Inserting icons from PowerPoint

The slide looks better; the next step is adding icons.

To insert an icon, go to the **Insert** tab and select Icons. The stock gallery will open with the icons displayed. Type in a search term and see if you can find a suitable icon.

You may need to try a variety of search terms when looking for icons. Of course, it makes sense to start with keywords from your primary message text, but if you don't find what you want, don't be afraid to try another descriptive term. We used the search words "meeting", "path", and "process" to find the three icons we'll add to the slide.

Once the icons are on the slide, resize them just as you would other objects; press Shift to constrain the aspect ratio or use the size inputs on the ribbon.

Then you can drag them into place. As with other objects, Smart Guides will appear to help you centre the icons to the boxes. You will learn about alignment tools in Chapter 9.

Changing the icon colour

To change the icon colour, select one or all of the icons and use **Graphics Format** > Graphics Fill to choose bright blue or another colour. With the stock PowerPoint icons, changing the fill colour changes the icon colour, even if they appear to be outlined shapes (Figure 7.17).

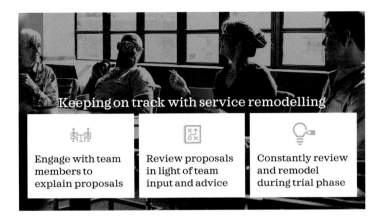

Figure 7.17 Our final slide with bright blue icons to support each of the three key messages.

Other sources of icons

There are, of course, other sources of icons, which we discussed in Chapter 4. Usually you'll download the icon and insert it onto your slide using **Insert** > Pictures > This Device. If the icon you insert is a vector format (SVG), you can recolour it using the tools on the **Graphics Format** tab, just like with PowerPoint stock icons. (Although occasionally you'll need to use **Graphics Format** > Graphics Outline in addition to Graphics Fill to recolour some of them.) If the icons are in raster format (PNG or JPEG), you'll need to use the **Picture Format** tools on the icon images.

The Noun Project has add-ins for both Mac and Windows that will let you search its icons from directly within PowerPoint, or you can go to their website and download icons there. (The add-in is super convenient!)

You should know that colour is applied differently to raster images and vector graphics. Because of this, our recommendation is to use the same file format for your icons—either all vector (SVG) or all raster (PNG or JPEG)—because it will be easier for you to match their colours, making them look more cohesive overall.

CONCLUSION

Adding images and icons is a fantastic way to reduce the amount of text needed on your slides. Carefully chosen images can significantly enhance your message and make your talk memorable.

8

Inserting logos and crests

When you present at a meeting, whether using slides or a poster, you may want to include some logos or crests. These may be for your own institution, to credit a source of support, or they may be the logo of the meeting itself. Some institutions use crests rather than logos. For the purposes of this chapter, we will use the term logo for both.

LESS IS MORE

The first question you should ask is: Do you really need to add these logos? Don't put them in just for show; they must be relevant.

If you do feel the need to add logos, try to restrict the number. They need space to breathe, so don't squash too many in together and don't fill the whole slide with them. This just looks cluttered and untidy. If multiple logos are used, be sure to align them accurately (see Chapter 9) and size them to match each other.

The next question is where should you put the logos? As a rule, you can safely add them to the title slide and/or the final slide. There is rarely any need to include logos on every slide; they will use up valuable space and your slide content may overlap them. Furthermore, logos on every slide are a distraction. Remember cognitive load?

If you use section divider slides, you might include a logo there.

If you apply a stock theme in PowerPoint, don't place your logo or crest over the background graphics. If necessary, switch off the background graphics on individual slides from the **Design** tab (Format Background > Hide Background Graphics).

Remember, less is more. You don't want lots of distracting elements cluttering your slides.

DOI: 10.1201/9781003287902-10

Style guidelines

Most academic institutions will have a website with style guidelines. Here you will find files for logos and crests. In addition, the style guidelines will often tell you how best to display these elements.

WHICH IMAGE FILE TYPE?

In Chapter 4 we explained the different types of images. You will recall that raster images have a fixed size (resolution). If you must use a raster image such as a PNG or JPEG, try to find a high-resolution version. If your raster image is low resolution, when you enlarge it, it may pixelate.

If a vector format of the logo is available, use it. Vectors usually have transparent backgrounds, they can be scaled to different sizes without quality loss and they can easily be recoloured. SVG is the easiest because you can insert it directly into PowerPoint using **Insert** > Pictures > Picture From File.

Unfortunately, although they are scalable, encapsulated postscript (EPS) images are not supported by PowerPoint, so you can't use them directly. However, you can convert an EPS logo to an SVG, PNG, or JPEG using the online converter at cloudconvert.com

With any logo, as with any image or shape, resize it by dragging from the corner to maintain its aspect ratio and prevent distortion.

TRANSPARENCY

Like SVGs, PNG images support transparency and can be placed on a coloured background. This is great if you have a coloured slide background (Figure 8.1)!

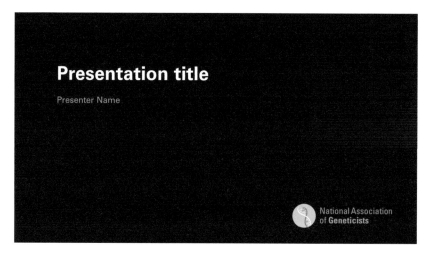

Figure 8.1 A logo with a transparent background looks great on a coloured slide.

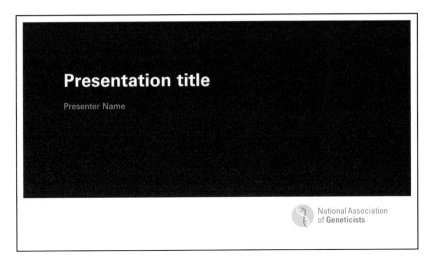

Figure 8.2 **A JPEG will be surrounded by a white box, so place it on a white background.**

If you use a JPEG on a coloured background, you will see a white box surrounding the logo. For this reason, we recommend that you always place JPEGs on a white area of your slide. If your slide is not white, a simple way to do this is to place a white rectangle across the whole of the bottom of the slide and all your logos can sit here (Figure 8.2).

Removing the background of a logo

PowerPoint has a tool for removing the background from raster images. To use it, click on the image, then in the **Picture Format** tab, select Remove Background. By all means try this, but it is not particularly accurate, and you will often end up with a rather ragged edge to the image. Dropping out a background is much better done in an image editor such as Photoshop or online tools such as remove.bg.

RECOLOURING A LOGO

One reason we like vector logos is because they are easy to recolour. Of course, you'll want to double-check the brand guides to make sure the institution allows this, but it's fairly common to permit a logo to be coloured white for dark backgrounds or black for light backgrounds. To recolour an SVG logo, select it and choose a colour from **Graphics Format** > Graphics Fill.

Recolouring raster graphics is more difficult; we don't recommend it. However sometimes, it is possible to turn a raster logo white or black by adjusting the brightness and contrast settings in the **Picture Format** > Corrections > Picture Corrections Options tools.

CONCLUSION

Adding a logo or crest to your slide is a great way to acknowledge support for your work. However, use discretion and limit the number of logos to avoid slide clutter. Be sure to follow the instructions in Chapter 9 regarding the alignment and spacing of slide elements. Try to avoid logos overlapping the slide background graphics.

Don't place a logo on every slide. Restrict them to the title and perhaps the concluding slides.

Finally the safest choice for most logos is to place them on a white background.

9

Alignment and grouping objects on your slides

A skilled clinician has an innate feel for what is both right and wrong with a patient. However, this is only part of the story; this innate skill is complemented by meticulous attention to detail in the history, examination, laboratory investigation and imaging.

There are similarities in presentation design. We all recognise good design, even if we don't know why it is good. An impactful presentation requires both a feel for general design principles as well as attention to detail, such as accurate alignment and sympathetic colour choices. Trust us on this one—people may not notice when your content is perfectly aligned, but they will definitely notice when it is not. This can be the difference between an ordinary presentation and a great one.

In this chapter, we will guide you through a few suggestions that will elevate your slide design to a higher level, even though you are not a designer.

ALIGNING WITH SMART GUIDES

Probably the easiest way to align objects in PowerPoint is by using the Smart Guides. Smart Guides are the orange lines that appear when you're dragging an object around on your slide. They indicate when objects' sides, middles and centres are aligned. For example, when you're centring objects to each other, you'll see a "crosshair" similar to that pictured in Figure 9.1.

Smart Guides should be turned on in PowerPoint by default. If they're not, right-click in an empty area of the slide, click the arrow next to Grid and Guides, and select Smart Guides to toggle them on.

ALIGNING WITH ALIGNMENT TOOLS

Smart Guides will get you where you need to be 95% of the time. For the other 5%, you can use PowerPoint's alignment tools. These let you align objects by the left or right side, the top or bottom edge, or the vertical centre or horizontal middle.

DOI: 10.1201/9781003287902-11

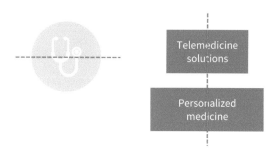

Figure 9.1 Smart Guides will help you align objects, such as when you're centring an icon on top of a circle or aligning two shapes or text boxes.

The important thing to know here is that PowerPoint will align all the selected objects to the most extreme edge available. For example, if you have a group of shapes selected, and you choose **Home** > Arrange > Align > Align Bottom, PowerPoint will use the object with the bottommost edge as the "anchor" and move all other selected objects to align with that edge. If you choose Align Right, then PowerPoint will use the object with the rightmost edge as the anchor to align to. And so on.

When you are aligning the centre or middle, PowerPoint will split the difference and move both objects. The exception is if one object is smaller than the other(s); in that case, PowerPoint will use the largest object as the anchor.

Alignment tools are available on the **Home** tab as well as various contextual tabs such as **Shape Format** and **Picture Format**. And yes, we know there are many layers to go through before you can select the alignment tool you want! For this reason, we added the alignment tools to our Quick Access Toolbar for quick and easy access. Refer to Chapter 5 for more information on setting up your QAT (Figure 9.2).

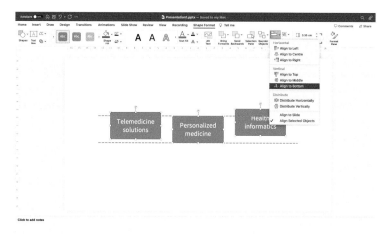

Figure 9.2 Use the alignment tools to align selected objects to a side or centre of objects. Here, where we've opted to Align bottom, the two boxes on the sides will be moved lower to Align with the bottom edge of the box in the middle.

DISTRIBUTING OBJECTS

Distribution refers to the space between objects, and you can use the Smart Guides and the Alignment tools to help distribute objects equally.

When you drag objects around on the slides, you'll see the alignment guides discussed above, and you'll also see the distribution arrows, as pictured in Figure 9.3. Not only will the distribution Smart Guides indicate when your objects are equidistant from each other, but they'll often show you when the objects are the same distance from the edges of the slide.

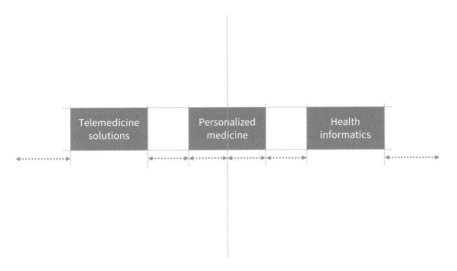

Figure 9.3 Smart Guides will appear as arrows to help you distribute objects on your slides.

If you prefer to use the Alignment tools—and sometimes that's easier, especially if there are a ton of objects on your slide, which can make the Smart Guides a little overwhelming—select the objects you want to distribute and choose **Home** > Arrange > Align > Distribute Horizontally. PowerPoint will use the leftmost object for the left anchor and the rightmost for the right anchor, and it will reposition any objects between the two. (Of course, if you're distributing vertically, PowerPoint will use top and bottom anchor points instead of left and right.) Note that this means you'll need to choose at least three items to distribute – one for the left or topmost, one for the right or bottommost, and then any others for the in-between.

ALIGNING AND DISTRIBUTING TO THE SLIDE

Sometimes you'll want to align or distribute objects on the slide overall. To do this, choose **Home** > Arrange > Align > Align to Slide, then align or distribute as usual. When you turn on Align to Slide, PowerPoint uses the edges of the slide as your left, right, top, and bottom anchors and then aligns or distributes the selected objects to that.

Once you've finished distributing the objects to the slide, don't forget to go back and choose **Home** > Arrange > Align > Align Selected Objects to turn off the Align to Slide setting (Figure 9.4).

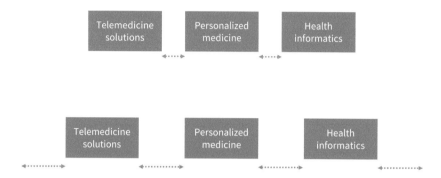

Figure 9.4 Boxes on the top have been distributed horizontally using Align Selected Objects. Boxes on the bottom have been distributed horizontally with Align to Slide selected.

If you select only one object and choose an Align or Distribute option, PowerPoint will assume that you meant to choose Align to Slide and will activate that setting automatically.

GROUPING OBJECTS CAN HELP WITH ALIGNMENT

What if you've painstakingly aligned a bunch of text boxes on your slide but then you realise the whole thing is off-centre? Don't worry! You don't have to start over!

You already know that aligning or distributing one object automatically engages the Align to Slide setting. Well, grouping your objects together will make them act as one. You can use this to your advantage!

For example, don't be afraid to select all the objects on your slide, group them together (Ctrl + G (Windows) or ⌘ + Option + G (Mac), and choose **Home** > Arrange > Align > Align Centre to centre the entire set on the slide.

In fact alignment is best accomplished in steps, often interspersing grouping and ungrouping as needed. We frequently align two or three objects—an icon and the shape behind it is common—and then group them together. This makes it easy to use the Smart Guides or alignment tools to align the "icon shape" with other objects on the slide (Figure 9.5).

Once you've aligned the icon shape and any related label text boxes, you can group all of them together, select the group, and press Ctrl [⌘] + D to duplicate

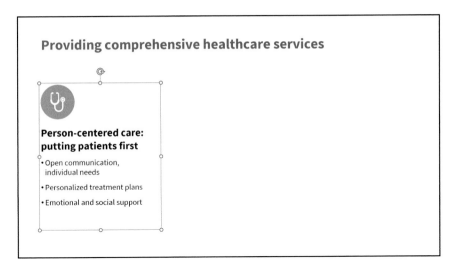

Figure 9.5 Alignment and distribution usually happen in steps. Here the icon and circle were aligned and then grouped. Then the text boxes were left-aligned with the icon group.

it. When you drag it into place, the Smart Guides will help ensure everything's aligned (Figure 9.6).

Once the duplicate is in place, before you do anything else, press Ctrl [⌘] + D again to create another duplicate—and it will be placed in the proper position, as though the three groups had been distributed already! But as you can see in

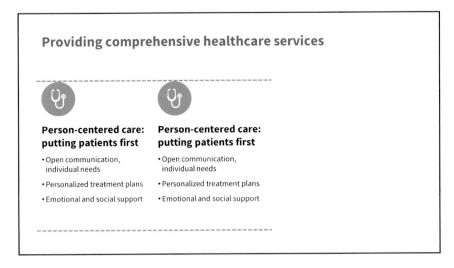

Figure 9.6 Alignment and distribution usually happen in steps. Next the icon and text boxes were grouped together and duplicated. Dragging them on the slide will activate the Smart Guides to help with alignment.

Providing comprehensive healthcare services

Person-centered care: putting patients first

- Open communication, individual needs
- Personalized treatment plans
- Emotional and social support

Person-centered care: putting patients first

- Open communication, individual needs
- Personalized treatment plans
- Emotional and social support

Person-centered care: putting patients first

- Open communication, individual needs
- Personalized treatment plans
- Emotional and social support

Figure 9.7 Alignment and distribution usually happen in steps. Here we have three groups, but they're not well placed on the slide.

Figure 9.7, the three objects aren't necessarily placed well on the slide in general. This is where we'd select all three groups and group them together. Then choose **Home** > Arrange > Align > Align Centre to centre them on the slide itself.

If you want, you can ungroup all the objects to edit them. In this example we have groups within groups—which you might call nested groups—so you'll be pressing Shift + Option + [⌘] + G, Shift + Ctrl + G a lot! Or you can click on any object within the group to alter it, which makes it simple to edit and format text, especially.

Providing comprehensive healthcare services

Person-centered care: putting patients first

- Open communication, individual needs
- Personalized treatment plans
- Emotional and social support

Advanced medical technology

- Cutting-edge technology
- Latest procedures
- Less invasive, more efficient treatments

Community engagement: promoting wellness

- Promoting community health and wellness
- Health events, education, preventative care
- Engaging with the community, promoting healthy behaviors, improving population health

Figure 9.8 Alignment and distribution usually happen in steps. Grouping all objects on the slide so they act as one object makes it easier to align everything to the slide as a whole.

If you're using the stock Microsoft icons, you can even right-click on the icons and choose Change Graphic > From Icons to swap them out without ungrouping.

Note: If you are a button rather than a shortcut person, there is an Ungroup option in the Arrange button on the **Home** tab.

PICTURE ALIGNMENT

We covered pictures a couple of chapters ago, but for some reason, slides with headshots have some of the worst alignment we see (Figure 9.9a,b)!

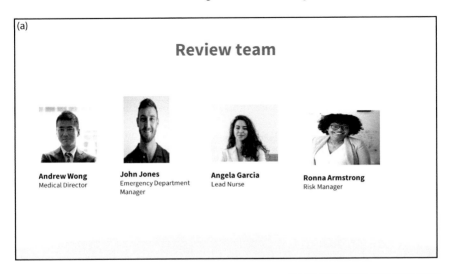

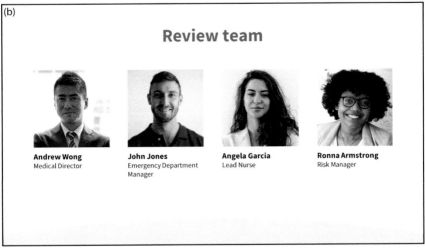

Figure 9.9 We often see slides like this (a) with extremely poor alignment. Correcting the image distortion and alignment doesn't take long to make a much more professional slide (b).

We want to point out a few things with this team slide because things like this make your slides look really unprofessional.

First is, of course, the images. We know you'll sometimes get cell phone images and downloaded pictures instead of professional headshots, but that's no excuse for squashed or stretched pictures! You can start by choosing an image and selecting **Picture Format** > Reset Picture > Reset Picture and Size. This will correct any distortion, and if the image is large, it may become huge! That's okay; you know that you can drag the corner or input an appropriate size in the Size area of the Picture Format tab to make it fit on the slide.

Once you've reset the picture to a size you can manage, crop it to a 1:1 aspect ratio for a square image or use one of the built-in portrait aspect ratios. This makes it super easy to crop all the images to the same aspect shape! For a refresher on cropping to aspect ratio, see Chapter 7.

Next is the text. You'll probably want to create a bit of a hierarchy with the text by making the names bigger and bolder and the titles a bit smaller and less prominent.

Of course, this is an alignment chapter, so we have to point out the poor alignment! When all the images are the same size, aligning them using either Smart Guides or the alignment tools will be easy. Don't forget to align the tops of the text boxes as well. And please! Take the time to group each headshot with its label so you can distribute them all on the slide.

BUILDING A CONSORT DIAGRAM

We can use the concepts you've learned in this chapter to create a nice, clean consort diagram (Figure 9.10).

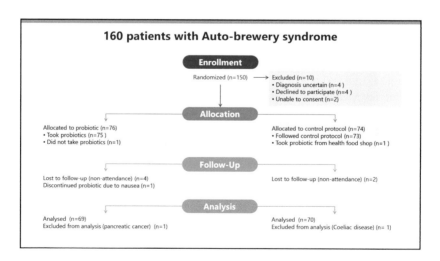

Figure 9.10 Our consort diagram is simply formatted and perfectly aligned, letting people focus on the content. Note also that the colour scheme is subtle.

The key to creating a clean study design like this is to remember that less is more. Resist the urge to add lots of colour-coding and formatting, and we promise you that your diagram will be better for it. It may also help to sketch the diagram before you start constructing it in PowerPoint. Having an idea of what you intend the diagram to look like can make it easier to create and eliminate a lot of false starts.

To create the main headings (enrolment, allocation, follow-up, and analysis), insert a rounded corner rectangle and drag the yellow adjustment handle to create the capsule shape you see here. Remove the shape outline, type and format the text, and then centre the shape on the slide.

Then duplicate the capsule shape using Ctrl [⌘] + D and drag it into place. If you immediately create two more duplicates in this manner, they will automatically be vertically spaced on the slide. You should be able to change the text and fill colours easily.

Next create the rectangle that gives additional information for each step. Format and size the first shape, filling it with the lightest tint of the colour used for the heading. Then drag the rectangle into its approximate place. Duplicate it as you did with the capsule shapes so that everything is in its approximate position. This is where it helps to have an idea of what the diagram will look like!

You could use elbow connectors to create the arrows, but we'll be honest—elbow connectors are fiddly and prone to collapsing, so we usually end up making our own. To create the arrows, draw a horizontal line, then draw a vertical arrow. You should be able to feel the arrow and the line fit together as you drag one close to the other. (Zooming in can sometimes help with that. Ctrl [⌘] + to zoom in and Ctrl [⌘] – to zoom out.) Once they're "connected", group the line and arrow, and you'll be able to drag the edges of the group to make them wider, narrower, taller or shorter.

Drag your "custom" elbow connector into place so it touches the edge of the heading capsule and points downward to the rectangle with the descriptive text. Drag the side of the connector to size it so the arrow is in the middle of the rectangle. A Smart Guide should appear to help you with this.

Once you have one elbow connector positioned, you can duplicate it and drag the copies into position. You can also use **Home** > Arrange > Rotate > Flip Horizontal to create the elbow connectors for the opposite side.

Add the text box for the N, and then finalise the diagram: Tweak the position of the various objects as needed, add the straight arrows from Enrolment to Allocation, change the arrowheads if you'd like, format the arrows to match the heading colour, etc. The truth is, you could create this diagram using black and grey shades, and it would be just as effective. The key here is in the clean formatting and perfect alignment.

10

Animations and transitions

We could summarise this chapter in one sentence. Less is more, and none is usually better!

What are animations and transitions and what is the difference?

WHAT'S THE DIFFERENCE?

Animations are effects applied to objects within a slide. Transitions are effects applied as one slide changes to the next, that is, effects between slides.

ANIMATIONS

Animation can be added to almost any slide content, but the most common objects to be animated are shapes and images.

Text rarely benefits from animation. Indeed text that flies in from the side or appears line by line can be profoundly irritating. Furthermore, evidence suggests that animating text creates unnecessary additional (extrinsic) cognitive load and reduces recall.[1] So our advice is only to animate text when there is a clear benefit for the viewer and not because you think it looks cool.

OPENING THE ANIMATIONS TAB

Clicking the **Animations** tab will open the animations tools. If you've not selected anything on the slide, the animations tools will be greyed out (Figure 10.1).

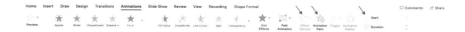

Figure 10.1 The animation tab, note the .three greyed out options.

 DOI: 10.1201/9781003287902-12

Starting with a blank slide, insert a rectangle as learnt in Chapter 6. You can add some text to the rectangle or change its colour if you wish. Select the rectangle, and you can see that animation options are now available. Objects have no animations by default, but you can easily add them.

Types of animation

There are four types of animation available: Entrance, Emphasis, Exit, and Motion Path. These can be combined or used in a sequence. You can also set the time that the animations take to complete.

As the name suggests, **Entrance animations** change how an object appears on the slide. For example, "Appear" makes the object immediately display, while "Fade" makes it appear more gradually.

Emphasis animations are used to add or remove emphasis to an object. For example, you can change text to bold or make a shape or text change colour.

Exit animations give you different ways to remove an object from a slide. For example, you can apply "Disappear" to immediately remove the object or use the "Fade" exit animation to let an object gradually disappear.

Motion Paths let you move an object from one position to another on the slide. Motion path animations are pretty advanced, but Morph transitions can be a good alternative.

To add an animation to an object, select it, then click one of the animations from the ribbon to apply. You will see a preview of the animation and the applied animation will be highlighted in the animation gallery.

Although animations animate identically on Mac and Windows, adding, changing, and applying multiple animation effects differ slightly on each platform. (It's probably easier to see what's happening if you open the animation pane while you're trying this out.)

On Mac, select an object, then click an animation in the gallery to apply it. If you don't like it, you can immediately click another animation to apply it *instead*. To apply a *second* animation effect, click away from the object to deselect it, then re-select the object and click another animation effect. Continue to click away and re-select the object to add more animations to the "stack".

On Windows, select the object and click an animation in the animation gallery to apply it. Click the Add Animation button to add a second animation to an object. Otherwise, if you choose from the main animations gallery (as you would on Mac PowerPoint), you will always overwrite the original animation with the new one.

Starting animations

Once you've added an animation to an object, you can specify how it starts. This lets you control whether the animations happen together or sequentially. These options are under Timing in the Animation Pane. You can also select them from the Start options on the Ribbon on the far-right side (Figure 10.2).

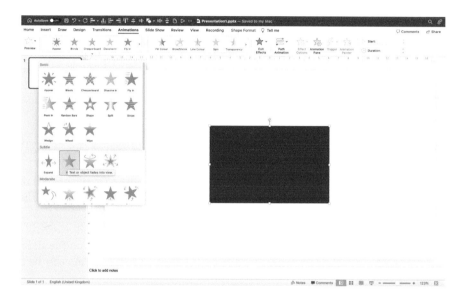

Figure 10.2 **Adding a simple Fade Animation.**

On Click will start the animation when you advance, whether that's by hitting the spacebar, using the arrows on the keyboard, clicking a button on a remote slide advancer (a "clicker"), clicking your mouse button, clicking the buttons in Presenter View, and so on. You would click to advance to the slide and then click again when you're ready to start the animation.

With Previous starts one animation at the same time as another animation or action. If there's only one animated object, "With Previous" will automatically start the animation when the slide starts. You would click to advance to the slide, then the animation would start automatically.

After Previous automatically starts one animation after the other animation finishes.

Once you've set up your animation, you can do a quick test by clicking the Preview button on the Animations tab. Better yet, review in Slide Show View to ensure everything works as expected.

OTHER ANIMATION SETTINGS AND TOOLS

You can also specify various effect options and settings for duration and delay.

Effect Options

The available Effect Options will depend on the animation that's been applied and the object it's been applied to. If you've added a simple Fade to text, you'll have options to animate the text all at once or by paragraph. If you've added a Wipe animation to a shape, you'll see options to animate from top, bottom, left, or right.

Animation duration and delay

Duration controls the time it takes for the animation to happen. For example, the Fade entrance animation duration is 0.5 seconds, but you can extend it to 2 seconds (or longer) for a slow fade.

Delay controls the time between the starting cue for an animation and when the animation actually begins. For example, if you want to click the mouse and have the animation begin 1 second later, you'd add a 1.00 delay to the animation. Delays are used mostly in very complex animation sequences. On Mac you'll need to open the Animation Pane, select the animation in the list, and then the Timings tab to access Delay settings.

Animation painter

You may want to apply the same animation to multiple objects on a single slide or even to objects on several slides. Rather than selecting each object and manually setting all the animation options again, there is a handy way to do this.

Select the object to which you have already applied the animation, then click Animation Painter on the **Animations** tab. Hover over the object you wish to apply the animation to, and when the cursor changes to a paintbrush, click on the object. Hey, presto! The animation and its settings are "painted" onto that object. This can save you a load of time and trouble.

If you want to apply the animation to multiple objects one after the other, double-click the Animation Painter button. The animation painter will stay enabled (you can see the paintbrush cursor); just click away on your desired objects, even across slides. Click the Animation Painter button again or hit Esc on your keyboard to disable this "sticky" mode.

Animation Pane

If you need more control over the animations than you see available to you in the Ribbon, click the Animation Pane button to open the Animation Pane (shown in

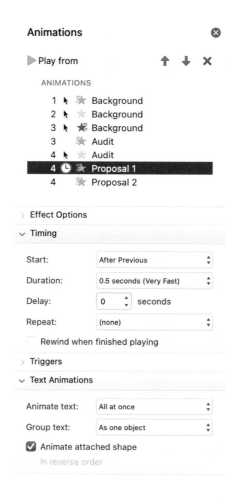

Figure 10.3 A complex series of Animations, seen in the Animation Pane (Mac).

Figure 10.3), where you have access to many more settings, most of which you'll never need!

On a Mac, when you select an animation in the list, you'll see the additional settings at the bottom of the pane. On Windows, you'll need to click the arrow to the right of the animation in the list to open a menu with the additional settings. On Windows, you can also see the animation timeline in the pane, which might help you visualise the order and timing of the animations.

You can click and drag or use the arrows at the top to reorder animations in the Animation Pane.

Figure 10.3 shows the construction of a complex series of animations. The arrows to the left of the first three animations for the background image (green Entrance: Fade, yellow Emphasis: Transparency and red Exit: Fade) indicate that these animations are on a series of clicks. The next animation (Audit) is an entrance animation. There is no icon next to it because it happens at the same time as the Previous animation (With Previous; the number 3 also indicates that it is part of the third animation set). The penultimate animation (Proposals1) has a clock face beside it, indicating that it occurs after the previous animation (and the final animation occurs with it).

Note that it is easier to see which animation is which when the objects are renamed in the Selection Pane.

Selection Pane

You will probably have noticed that it can be difficult to tell which object is which when they are given names like "Rectangle 2" by PowerPoint. You can rename objects in the Selection Pane so they're easier to distinguish. Enable the selection pane by selecting any object on the slide and then clicking **Home** > Arrange > Selection Pane. You can also enable the selection pane on many of the contextual tabs (**Shape Format**, **Picture Format**, etc.); just look for the Arrange tools, and the Selection Pane will be right there!

Once you open the Selection Pane, you can double-click on the names of objects and rename them, as shown in Figure 10.4. And if you rename objects in the Selection Pane, you can also see those names in the Animation Pane!

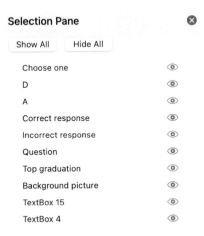

Figure 10.4 The Selection Pane. Objects can be renamed and the order changed by dragging them (this will change the order from front to back on the slide).

Triggers

Triggers are a more complex instruction to start a sequence of animations when you click on a specific object or area of a slide. Triggers aren't used often, but they can be super helpful for games and interactive presentations.

A simple example of a trigger effect would be to have a slide with a question and two possible answers. Clicking the correct answer will trigger the appropriate feedback box to animate in.

EXAMPLES OF ANIMATION TECHNIQUES

Now that you've got the lay of the land with the various animation options let's see some animation in action.

EXAMPLE 1: TEXT BOX (OR SHAPE) ENTERS ON CLICK

You are preparing some revision (study guides) for students and want them to address a series of questions. The goal is to have the text box with the answer appear when the slide is advanced (in other words, when the mouse is clicked) (Figure 10.5).

To set this up, select the answer text box and on the Animations tab, click Fade in the green entry animations. Leave everything else in the default settings. Now the answer will only reveal itself when the viewer is ready and clicks the mouse button or otherwise advances the slide.

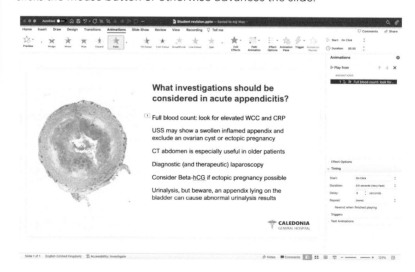

Figure 10.5 A Fade animation applied to the text box for the answer to the question in the title. (Image courtesy of Dr Maurice Loughrey.)

EXAMPLE 2: TEXT BOX OR SHAPE EXITS ON CLICK

You might have a similar slide where you want to remove a text box or object. Use an exit animation for that (Figure 10.6).

Set this slide up just as you did for the entrance animation (but with four separate text boxes) but select one of the red exit animations instead. In this example, the last text box will fade away when the slide is advanced, removing the one incorrect response.

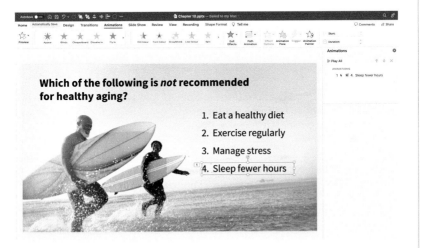

Figure 10.6 A simple fade exit animation of a text box containing the incorrect answer.

EXAMPLE 3: KEY MESSAGE ZOOMS IN, PICTURE FADES "WITH PREVIOUS"

A zoom entrance animation can emphasise your message nicely.

In this example, we have a screenshot of a (fictitious) journal article on the slide. We've added a text box with a semi-transparent white fill and large text to emphasise the article's key takeaway.

In this case, we want the article to be shown first when we present the slide so we can give a general overview of the study. Then when we click the mouse, we want the article to fade a bit and the key message to zoom in.

To set up this animation, select the screenshot of the article and choose Transparency from the yellow emphasis animations. To adjust it, open the Animation Pane and click on the transparency animation in the list.

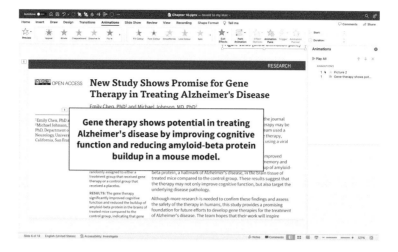

Figure 10.7 Setting up animations in PowerPoint for Mac. The background PDF is set to become semi-transparent, and at the same time, the text box enters with a zoom animation.

On Mac, click Effect Options at the bottom of the pane and change Property to 75%. On Windows, double-click the transparency animation in the pane and on the Effect tab in the dialogue, change the setting to 75% (Figure 10.7).

Next select the key message text box and apply the Zoom entrance animation. On the far right of the Animations tab, change the duration of the Zoom entrance to 1 second to slow it down a bit. Finally, change the start setting from On Click to With Previous so the text box will zoom in as the article image fades and you don't have to click multiple times for your animations to occur (Figure 10.8)!

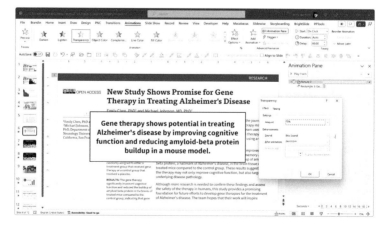

Figure 10.8 Setting up the same animation as Figure 10.7 in PowerPoint for Windows.

EXAMPLE 4: MULTIPLE ANIMATIONS ON ONE OBJECT

You can add more than one animation to any object on a slide. In this example, we've grouped text boxes together with a graphical rule line for some visual interest. Our goal is for only one group to be visible at a time. You could animate all of these objects individually, but it's easier and faster to animate three groups than six individual objects!

Begin by selecting the first group and adding a Fade entrance animation. By default, it will start on click (Figure 10.9).

Then add a Fade *exit* animation to the same group. Remember, to apply additional animations on Mac, deselect the object, then re-select it and select the animation from the main Animations gallery. On Windows, you can simply open the Add Animation gallery to apply multiple animations to an object. This second animation will also start on click.

Once you've added both animations to the group, either repeat the steps for the other two groups or use the animation painter to apply the animations from the first group to the second and third groups. In Figure 10.10, you can see how the start-on-click entrance and exit animations look in the Animation Pane at this point. Click once to make Group 1 animate in. Click again to make Group 1 fade out. Click again to make Group 2 animate in,

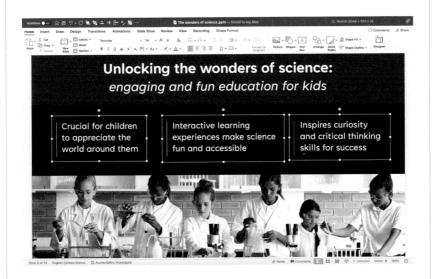

Figure 10.9 **Grouped objects to be animated in a sequence.**

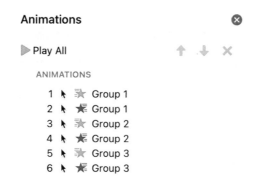

Figure 10.10 The animation pane shows the (default on click) entrance and exit animations for Group 1, then Group 2, then Group 3.

and then click a fourth time to make it fade out. And so on. This is way too many clicks to worry about when you're presenting!

Thinking through this animation, Group 1 should automatically become visible when you advance to this slide. Change the Group 1 animation start setting to With Previous to make it fade in automatically. That way you don't have to click to advance the slide and immediately click again to reveal the animated Group 1 text.

With the next animation Group 1 fades away when you click the mouse or otherwise advance the slide. Wouldn't it be nice if Group 2 could fade in at the same time? To accomplish this, change the animation start setting for Group 2 to With Previous so it fades in at the same time Group 1 fades out. Do the same for Group 3 so it fades in when you click to make Group 2 fade out.

Finally we suggest removing that final exit animation for Group 3 altogether. Otherwise, you'll have to click to make Group 3 fade away and then immediately click again to advance to the next slide. Why bother? Just select that last animation in the Animation Pane and press Delete on your keyboard to get rid of it (Figure 10.11).

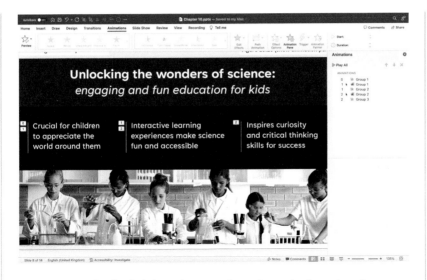

Figure 10.11 **The final slide with animations shown in the animation pane.**

A caution about animating grouped objects: you must animate the group itself. If you animate objects and then group them, the animation is deleted. Also any animation previously applied to that group is deleted if you ungroup.

EXAMPLE 5: TRIGGER ANIMATION

Triggers are excellent for creating games, interactive presentations, quizzes, and the like. To trigger an animation basically means, "Click this object to trigger another object to animate". It's really just another way to start an animation.

In this example we've created a quiz for students. When the student clicks each of the response circles, a rectangle with appropriate information appears, one to support the correct answer and one for the incorrect response (Figure 10.12).

To set up a trigger animation, first you have to animate the objects. In this case since the relevant feedback text boxes should animate in, add a fade entrance animation to each of the two boxes. It doesn't matter what start setting you specify for these because the trigger will replace it.

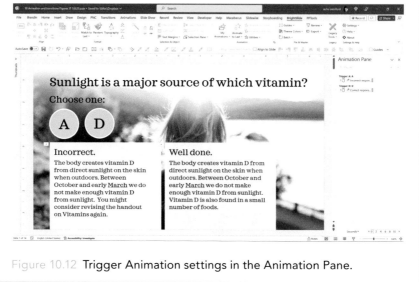

Figure 10.12 **Trigger Animation settings in the Animation Pane.**

Next set each feedback box to be triggered by the appropriate response. Select the "correct" feedback box, then click **Animations** > Trigger > On click of, and choose the "D" oval from the list. (It really helps to rename your objects in the Selection Pane if you plan to add trigger animations!) Now when the presenter clicks circle D, it will trigger the "correct" feedback box to animate in.

Do the same for the "incorrect" box, but of course, choose the "A" oval as the trigger. This will trigger the "incorrect" box to animate when clicking circle A.

EXAMPLE 6: MORPH TRANSITION

For 99% of all our presentations, we use a simple fade transition between all the slides. Why? The reason is simple: Transitions need to be subtle that the viewer isn't conscious that they are happening (with notable exceptions, see below). This reduces extraneous cognitive load. If you have no transition, the slides can be jarring as you move from one to the next, so a fade is a very good compromise.

Select a slide and click the **Transitions** tab. Choose the Fade transition and then on the far right of the ribbon, Apply to All. That's it, done!

There is, however, a new transition in Office 365 that can be really useful but must be used sparingly. This is the Morph transition. Morph transitions allow you to easily move or change an object as you move from one slide to another. Because of this, the Morph transition is almost more like an animation than a transition.

The key to using Morph is to use the same object on subsequent slides.

In the slides shown in Figures 10.13 and 10.14, we copy-pasted the first slide. Then we faded the image, adding a title and a chart to the duplicate. The circle was also repositioned and resized with a smaller font on the duplicate slide.

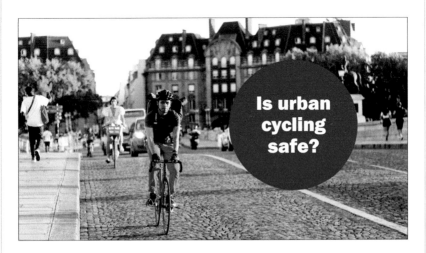

Figure 10.13 The first slide in a Morph sequence.

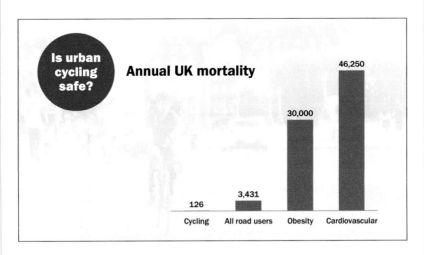

Figure 10.14 The second slide in a Morph sequence.

With a typical Fade transition, the first slide would appear and then the second slide would fade in with the circle in its new place. However, if you apply a Morph transition to slide 2, when you test in Slide Show View, you'll see the circle actually move and get smaller.

Because the slide was duplicated PowerPoint recognised the circle as being the same object, and it morphed into its new size and position as we expected. But sometimes when you copy and paste objects from one slide to the next, PowerPoint doesn't recognise them as the same, so the Morph transition doesn't work.

To get around this you can fool PowerPoint into thinking two objects are the same by using two exclamation points and giving them the same name in the Selection Pane. For example if PowerPoint didn't morph our two circles properly, we might name them !!GreenCircle on both slides. Using the two exclamation marks tells PowerPoint that these two circles should be considered the same object, so it should morph one circle into the other as it transitions from one slide to the next.

EXAMPLE 7: PAN TRANSITION FOR TIMELINES

One of the most useful diagrams in medicine is to show a timeline. But sometimes timelines can be extremely complex and crowded. To better display your timeline, consider spreading it over a few separate slides and using a Pan transition to move it along.

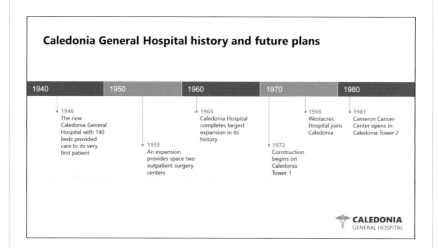

Figure 10.15 An example timeline spread over two slides.

A Pan transition lets the background graphics at the slide layout level stay still while other content (in this case the timeline) moves. In the selection pane, rename any objects that you don't want to move using the !! technique. For example, if you want the slide title to remain static, open the selection pane and rename the title to !!Title in both slides.

Then select Pan from the Transitions gallery on the second slide, and then choose From Right in the Effect Options (Figure 10.16).

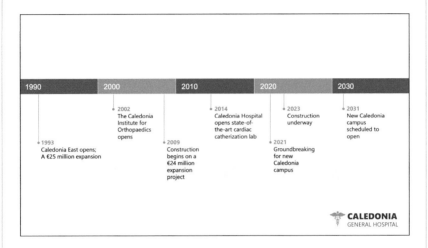

Figure 10.16 Using a Pan transition moves the timeline along while the background graphics (such as the logo) stay static.

CONCLUSION

Remember, fancy animations and transitions do not enhance your message, so it is important not to overuse these. It may seem cool when you first learn how to use animations and transitions, but the aim is to keep your audience focussed on your message, not your PowerPoint skills.

NOTE

1. Moreno R and Mayer RE *J Educ Psychol* 94, 156–163: 2002.

11

Inserting videos

In our workshops one of the most common issues that participants raise relates to using videos in PowerPoint. They are unsure of how to source videos and are afraid to use them based on past experience.

The risks associated with using video in PowerPoint have diminished significantly with recent versions. Previously, videos were linked to your presentation, so you had to save the video in the same folder as your talk before inserting it into the PowerPoint file.

In Microsoft 365 videos are embedded in the presentation and will travel with it wherever you take it. All you have to do is insert the video, and it will be embedded into PowerPoint by default.

VIDEO FILE FORMATS

There are a number of potential sources of video. You may have recorded the video yourself, or your medical photography team may have made it. Perhaps you have a video file from an endoscopy, radiology or minimal access procedure.

Microsoft 365 supports multiple video formats. However, .mp4 using an H.264 codec is the most compatible format and most likely to play whether you're on Mac or Windows, so we recommend that you stick with it.

INSERTING A VIDEO FILE FROM YOUR COMPUTER

If you have a video file that you want to include in your slide deck, begin by preparing the slide where you want to insert the video. We recommend a blank slide if your video will be played full screen. Of course, you may decide to play the video in only a part of the screen in some circumstances, and we will deal with that shortly.

Now choose **Insert** > Video > From File (to use a file on your computer) or Stock (to use a stock Microsoft video). Navigate to your video and click Insert. The

 DOI: 10.1201/9781003287902-13

video will appear on the slide and automatically be embedded in the PowerPoint file.

It is possible to link to a video instead of embedding it. This saves file size but can be extremely problematic, and we don't recommend it.

You may want the video to play full screen. If so, it doesn't matter what size the thumbnail of the video is at this stage. Simply select Play Full Screen from the **Playback** tab.

If you want the video to play in only part of the slide, you can adjust its dimensions as with any shape by simply dragging any corner of the thumbnail. If you drag from a corner, you do not need to worry about distortion, as the aspect ratio is automatically locked.

STARTING THE VIDEO

When you insert a video into your presentation from a file on your computer, by default, it's set up to play "In click sequence". This means the same as "on mouse click" in the animation settings, where the video will play as you advance the slide, whether by mouse click, space bar, arrow keys, or various other means.

You can set the video to play automatically, so you don't have to manually start it. Select your video and choose from the Start options on the **Playback** tab (Figure 11.1).

If you have a video such as an echocardiogram you also may want to tick "loop until stopped" on the **Playback** tab. This will play the video in a continuous loop.

Perhaps you need to stop the video to emphasise a particular area. You can pause and restart the video by clicking on it with the cursor (the cursor will change to a small hand). The right arrow or return key will move to the next slide.

You can place text boxes or shapes containing text over your video if you feel this adds to the message. Just be sure to add them after you add the video to ensure they are in front of the video or bring them to the front using the commands learnt in Chapter 6.

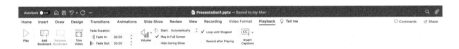

Figure 11.1 Once a video has been inserted, use the **Playback** tab to set the play options.

EDITING THE VIDEO

You may need to trim the beginning and end of your video. Select the video, and on the **Playback** tab, click Trim Video, then drag the sliders to your preferred start and finish points. Unfortunately, you can't trim out parts in the middle of the video in PowerPoint; you will need a video editing programme for that.

It is possible to adjust the volume of your video using the Volume button on the Playback tab. If your video has sound, remember to turn on your speakers in the operating system, too!

FORMATTING THE VIDEO

Video can be formatted in the same way as an image. You can add shadows, reflections and outlines and even rotate and crop the video. However, these changes won't affect a video showing in full screen mode, and in our experience, these embellishments don't add anything to the viewer's experience, so we'd discourage you from using them.

OPTIMISING FOR COMPATIBILITY

If you're working in Windows, PowerPoint has a handy feature to optimise the compatibility of videos. Go to **File** > Info, and if there are videos in your file, you may have the option to Optimize Media Compatibility to help improve compatibility when played on other devices.

You may also have an option to Compress Media in this same area. This is especially good to do if your files have become very large because of embedded video. You can choose from Standard, HD, or Full HD quality when you choose to compress.

No option built into PowerPoint can compress and optimise video on a Mac. There are third-party applications that can achieve this (including Handbrake), but these are beyond the scope of this book.

PLAYING MULTIPLE VIDEOS

On occasions you may want to play multiple videos at the same time on a single slide, for example, videos of endoscopy and radiology or multiple views from an echocardiogram. To do this, insert all your videos and position them on the slide. For all of the videos, set Start Automatically in the **Playback** tab.

Alternatively, open the **Animation** tab and then the Animation Pane. In the animation pane, highlight all the videos by holding down Shift as you select them. Then under Timing, select Start > With Previous.

ONLINE VIDEOS

Before using online videos, check the internet connection at your presentation venue. And remember, the bandwidth tends to get worse once the audience gets there!

What if you want to show a video that is online, such as on YouTube? You can use the commands **Insert** > Video > Online Movie (Mac) or **Insert** > Video > Online Video (Windows). Then insert the URL (the website details) for the YouTube video and click Insert. (You can get this from YouTube by clicking Share, which is currently found below the YouTube video, and then copy the URL.) This will insert the video onto the slide but note that online videos are not embedded into your presentation. PowerPoint only provides a link, and an online video will only play if you have a reliable, speedy internet connection when you are showing your presentation.

Furthermore, online videos will not give you the option in the **Playback** menu to play full screen. You need to drag the corners of the video to the corners of the slide if you want that to happen.

If you want to force YouTube to play the video without the thumbnails on the right side, try this: copy the YouTube link, then insert it into PowerPoint as above; however, after the word "watch" in the URL, insert _popup.

Compare these two links or try this with a YouTube link of your choice:

* https://www.youtube.com/watch?v=JZ7Cu6i7j4E
* https://www.youtube.com/watch_popup?v=JZ7Cu6i7j4E

What if you want to start partway through an online video? To do this on YouTube, pause the video at the point where you want to start playing. Then right-click on the video timeline on YouTube and select Copy Video URL At Current Time from the menu options. Use this URL when you insert the online movie into PowerPoint.

COPYRIGHT

Most online videos including those on YouTube are copyrighted. The YouTube terms and conditions specifically state that you may not download the content. Furthermore, video creators have invested time and money in producing videos and it is unreasonable to expect them to let you use their videos for free. If you are a YouTube Premium subscriber, you can save videos on your computer to watch later; however, this is intended for personal use.

Your best option if you want to show a YouTube video in your presentation is to contact the owner of the video and ask permission to show it. There are third-party applications and websites to download YouTube videos, but considering the copyright issues, we urge you to be very cautious about using these unless you believe the "Fair Use" law[1,2] applies.

Many medical societies have videos on their websites. You may well be able to use these for teaching, but read the terms and conditions carefully first.

VIDEO WON'T PLAY!

We rarely see issues lately with video not playing in PowerPoint. Microsoft has done a lot of work in this area, and it shows!

Remember, online videos are linked, not embedded into your presentation. If your online video doesn't play, it could be an issue with the available bandwidth—you need a pretty good connection in order to stream online video effectively.

If you don't have an option to play full screen, it's also because you've inserted an online video. You would need to download the video and use **Insert** > Video > From File in order to use this setting.

Additionally, if you linked to a video, even if it's on your computer, the video must be available, and the link must not be broken for it to play.

If you are on a Windows computer, the best way to ensure against these issues is to run the Optimize Compatibility tool in **File** > Info.

CONCLUSION

To sum up, video works much better in Microsoft 365 than most users believe, but there are significant copyright issues that you must consider. Nonetheless, video is a great teaching medium, and the effort of learning how to use video in your presentations is worthwhile.

NOTES

1. For UK see: https://tinyurl.com/ycxsxrkh
2. For US see: https://en.wikipedia.org/wiki/Fair_use

12

Saving and printing your presentation

It may seem odd that we would devote a whole chapter to these topics, but this is a relatively short chapter, and most users are not aware of the important options that are available.

SAVING YOUR PRESENTATION

OK, first off, get in the habit of saving your presentation regularly as you make edits. Nothing is worse than working on a slide deck for hours, only for your computer to crash.

SAVE YOUR FILE!

To save your file on your computer, choose **File** > Save As. Give it a name.

After that, you can save your file using **File** > Save. Or get into the habit of using Ctrl [⌘] + S frequently so you don't lose any of your hard work.

AUTOSAVE

If you have a connected online (virtual) drive such as One Drive or SharePoint Online, AutoSave automatically saves your file in real time to that virtual drive as you work—just as you would save the file manually—so that you don't have to worry about saving on the go. If you are working on a document saved online, turning on Autosave will ensure changes are saved to the online document so that collaborators can see your revisions almost in real time.

If you want to save your file with a new name, simply select **File** > Save As.

If you really need to get back to a previous edit, you can always access previously saved versions (even if the file name is unchanged). How you do this depends on which virtual drive you are using; a quick search online will tell you how to do

DOI: 10.1201/9781003287902-14

this for your preferred setup. For Microsoft One Drive log in to your Microsoft 365 account at www.office.com. Open the PowerPoint File and select "Saved to One Drive" on the orange bar at the top and then "Version History".

AUTORECOVER

Autorecover attempts to recover files in the event of an application or system crash. It does this by periodically saving a copy of the file *on your computer.* By default, Autorecover saves a recovery file every 10 minutes.

In Windows, the option is found by selecting **File** > Options > Save (Figure 12.1).

On a Mac, click on the word "PowerPoint" just to the right of the Apple symbol on the top-level menu and then Select Preferences or use the shortcut ⌘ -, (that's Command, minus and comma) holding down all three keys simultaneously (shortcuts can be horrible) and then select the Save button.

Tick Autorecover and use the arrows to set a suitable interval. We recommend saving every ten minutes.

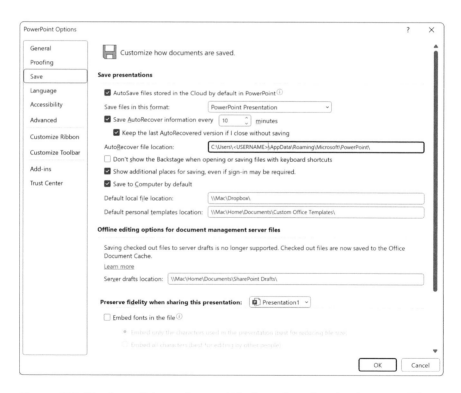

Figure 12.1 The Save dialogue box on Windows, found under the menu **File** > Options > Save.

FONT EMBEDDING

You'll also see options for Font Embedding at the bottom of this Save dialogue box (see Figure 12.2). This might seem like a good idea when using unusual fonts, but in reality, it's not that simple! There are several reasons why we don't recommend embedding fonts. We suggest you stick to the safer fonts listed in Chapter 13.

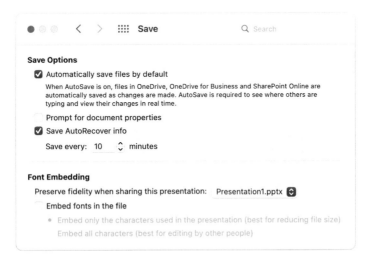

Figure 12.2 The Save dialogue box on a Mac found under the menu PowerPoint > Preferences > Save.

For starters, when you choose to embed fonts in the file, PowerPoint will embed *all* fonts in the presentation. Sometimes you'll have fonts you didn't know about. Fonts get introduced with copy-pasted content and can hide in speaker notes and the spaces between words. More fonts equal larger file sizes.

Also not all fonts can be embedded due to licensing restrictions. PowerPoint doesn't always warn you that a font is not embeddable when you save a file. And when someone else opens that file, they'll see a "read only" message and won't be able to edit or save on their end.

If you must use an unusual font in your presentation and want to be sure that font looks the same on another computer, try saving it as a PDF. See more on that later in this chapter.

SPECIFIC FILE TYPES FOR SAVING PRESENTATIONS

Normally when you save a PowerPoint file in Microsoft 365 it is saved as a .pptx file.

Saving as a PPTX

This file format was first introduced in Office versions dating back to Office 2007. It is an open XML standard (hence the x at the end of the old .ppt notation. Prior to 2007 PowerPoint files had the suffix .ppt), which means it can be opened using other programmes, including Open Office, Google Slides and Keynote.

The .pptx file is the one you will be most familiar with, and when you open it, it will usually open on Normal View, ready to edit.

Files saved in Microsoft 365 will retain their formatting and most of the newer features of PowerPoint, even if shown using older versions.

Saving as a PowerPoint Show – PPSX

You may want the convenience of a PowerPoint file that opens as a presentation and does not require you to go through "Normal View". Double-click the file in Finder or Windows Explorer; it opens in Slide Show View on the first slide, and off you go with your talk. This can look very slick. Furthermore, your audience will not see your slide thumbnails before you start your presentation.

To save this type of file, choose **File** > Save As > PowerPoint Show. This will be a .ppsx file.

If you need to edit the .ppsx file later, don't double-click it to open. Instead, choose **File** > Open in PowerPoint, navigate to the file, and click Open. This will open the .ppsx in Normal View. When you save it again, you need to decide whether to save it as a .pptx or a .ppsx file.

Saving as PowerPoint template

A .potx file is a PowerPoint template. When you double-click a POTX, the operating system opens a new file based on the template and leaves the original template file alone. This way your template file remains intact, and you don't inadvertently mess it up. Some online tools such as Dropbox, SharePoint, and OneDrive will open POTX files directly (and some won't open them at all), so it's perfectly fine to use a PPTX as your "template". Either way, keeping a copy of the file in your back pocket is always good.

We discuss PowerPoint templates in more detail in Chapter 14.

Saving as a PDF

It can be useful to have a backup of your presentation as a printed and/or electronic PDF (Portable Document Format). You can open and project this PDF and it will look for all the world like a PowerPoint show, except that there will be no animations or transitions.

This is your last-ditch backup plan if your presentation files fail you—believe us when we warn you that this does happen!

A PDF is also a great way to share a presentation when you want someone to review it but don't want to let them edit it (and mess up all your work).

Curiouser and curiouser!

The world of PDF files is strange, and we spent a while trying to make sense of this for you; we don't want to take you down a techie rabbit hole here, but sometimes creating a PDF file will hugely enlarge your file size for no apparent reason.

This isn't an issue for Windows users; just use the command sequence **File** > Export > Create PDF/XPS Document > Create PDF.XPS.

On a Mac it is more complex. Using the Mac native PDF creation tools sometimes results in very bloated files, and your PDF may not look as you intended, particularly if you use gradients or transparency.

Try using **File** > Export and in the dialogue box type a file name. Ensure the file format is PDF and then click Export. Be sure to carefully check the result—is the file high enough quality and a reasonable size? (To check the file size on a Mac, select **File** > Properties in Finder.)

If exporting the file to PDF using the native Mac PDF creation tool results in a poor-looking or bloated file, you can use a workaround to force PowerPoint to use its native PDF creation tools. Assuming you have a Microsoft 365 account—and you will, if you have a Microsoft 365 account—first save your presentation to OneDrive by making sure that Autosave is turned on. Then in your browser, go to www.office.com and log in to your Microsoft 365 account. Open the presentation from the One Drive. Now choose **File** > Save As > Download As PDF > Download. The PDF file will be saved to your downloads folder. You can then move it as required.

PRINTING YOUR PRESENTATION

Why on earth would you print a presentation? There are a few reasons:

- As a hard copy backup, in case the IT system fails. You can then hand out copies to attendees.
- As an aide memoire for you to practice your presentation without a computer (you can, of course, use PowerPoint on a smartphone for this).

- To have beside you as you present so that you know which slide numbers are which (but Presenter View is better).
- To print a handout. Many people print these with three slides and space to write notes on each page. In our experience, these are rarely of much value to the recipient. In fact they are not really a handout at all; they are a copy of your slides with room to write comments. You can do better by following the recommendations in Chapter 20.

To print the presentation from Normal view, select **File** > Print, or use the short-cut Ctrl [⌘] + P. You can then select your printer, choose paper size and orientation, and determine if you want to print some or all your slides. However, the most important choice is what layout to use.

You can print each slide on a single page—but what if you have 50 slides? You could print the default PowerPoint "handouts" with two, three, four, six or nine slides per page. The only one of these we would recommend is nine slides per page so that you can use this as an aide memoire during your talk. You should print in landscape setting for best results.

Most users will not want to print their presentation, but it is always good to know how in case the need arises.

13

Choosing fonts

Your audience should be able to easily read all the text on your slides. Choosing the right font can help you achieve this!

WHAT TO LOOK FOR WHEN SELECTING A FONT

Legibility is the most important visual characteristic of presentation fonts. You'll want to choose fonts that are simple in design so that the letterforms are distinguishable at smaller sizes (consider chart labels or table figures).

You might be familiar with Arial or Calibri, two of the most commonly used fonts in PowerPoint. These fonts are quite legible as they feature clean and simple letterforms. They are also good examples of "sans serif" fonts, which have less variation than "serif" fonts (with extended features at the ends of character strokes). Sans serif fonts are the best choice for presentation body text as they're typically more legible in small sizes. Serif fonts can be reserved for titles or larger text.

Look for fonts with lining figures—those with uniform height and alignment. Lining figures are preferable for data labels and table figures. Non-lining figures (old-style) have varying character heights, making them more visually disruptive when used for a lot of numbers (Figure 13.1).

Lining figures   01234567890

Non-lining
(old-style) figures   01234567890

Figure 13.1 Lining figures are preferred for displaying numbers in presentations.

Fonts have personality

You can't go wrong with Arial or Calibri, but perhaps you're looking for something different. As you scroll through the font picker in PowerPoint you'll see plenty of interesting and eye-catching typefaces, each with its own unique personality. Fonts convey a feeling or a mood with their character styles and stroke weights. Strong or weak, clean or cluttered, professional or juvenile … Your font choice can make a difference in how your presentation content is received.

Create a few different types of slides with varying text sizes for use when selecting a new font. Duplicate these slides and change the font on each set so you can visually compare your choices. Does the font help convey the meaning of your text? Does the font personality match the tone or subject of your presentation (Figure 13.2)?

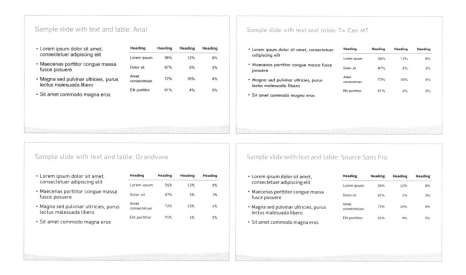

Figure 13.2 Sample slides can help you compare different fonts.

Choosing fonts for shared files

When you're creating a presentation that won't be shared beyond your computer, you can use any of the fonts on your system. However, most presentations *are* shared with others. When you share a .pptx file, you want to ensure that the fonts you've used won't be substituted on the receiving end. This can result in some messy-looking slides!

If you're working with an older version of PowerPoint (pre-Office 2019) or you're sharing your files with folks using an older version, it's best to stick with fonts that are already on their systems. Most everyone will have these classic fonts: Arial, Arial Black, Calibri, Cambria, Century Gothic, Franklin Gothic Book and Medium, Gill Sans MT, Rockwell, Tahoma, Trebuchet MS, Tw Cen MT, and Verdana.

If you and your colleagues are using newer versions of PowerPoint (Office 2019 or newer or Microsoft 365), you have many more choices. There are hundreds of new fonts available! These "cloud fonts" are designated by a cloud icon in the font picker. When selected for the first time, the font is automatically downloaded and placed in a separate folder on your system. You don't need to do anything; this download only occurs the first time you access the font. It can take a few seconds (or longer) for the new font to load and then you'll see it transform the text on your slide (Figure 13.3).

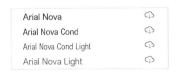

Figure 13.3 Cloud icons indicate fonts available for download.

There are many terrific new font families to choose from. Some of our favourites include: Avenir Next LT Pro, Daytona, Grandview, News Gothic MT, Seaford, Segoe UI, Source Sans Pro, Tenorite, and Trade Gothic Next. If you'd like to see other options, Julie has a visual guide to all of the cloud fonts: https://designto-present.com/2019/03/31/a-guide-to-cloud-fonts-in-microsoft-office-365/.

Note: If you'll be sharing presentations for a conference, it's safer to select one of the classic fonts listed above for use with older versions of Office. The conference computers might not have access to the internet, disabling the ability to download any newer fonts from the cloud.

Theme fonts

Ideally your font choices should be defined as the theme fonts (headings and body) within your template. These theme fonts will automatically populate all of the text in placeholders, charts, and shapes, helping you maintain a consistent look throughout your presentation. See the next chapter for details on setting up theme fonts.

Note: In 2023, Aptos was introduced as the new default font for the Microsoft 365 Office suite, replacing Calibri. In the new PowerPoint theme, Aptos Display is assigned as the Headings font and Aptos is the Body font.

14

Templates

PowerPoint has a terminology problem, and it's extremely noticeable when we start talking about templates. You may even be asking yourself, what is a PowerPoint template, exactly?

In PowerPoint parlance, a template is the underlying infrastructure of a file. You can think of it as the framework the slides are built on. A PowerPoint template includes a built-in set of theme fonts, theme colours and slide layouts. Every PowerPoint file includes these elements, whether you realise it or not.

The slide layouts are there to provide background graphics along with pre-positioned, pre-formatted placeholders for text and other content. The goal of a template is to save you time by streamlining some of the basic formatting and placement of text and other elements. A good template also helps create consistency throughout the file, which helps your presentation look more professional.

You are already familiar with the simplest templates shown in Figure 14.1.

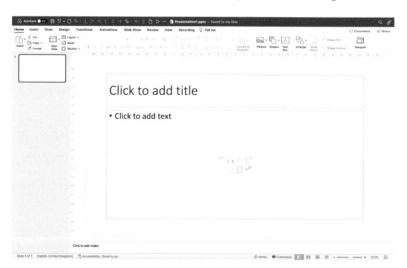

Figure 14.1 A blank slide with placeholders for a title and slide content.

DOI: 10.1201/9781003287902-16

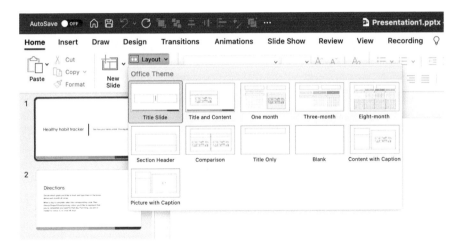

Figure 14.2 The Slide Layout gallery on a Mac shows one of the health-related themes available in Microsoft 365.

You can see the layouts in your file by expanding the New Slide gallery on the **Home** tab. To see the gallery on Mac, click the down arrow beside the New Slide button; on Windows, click the bottom of the New Slide button. If a layout you need isn't there, don't worry—keep reading, and you'll learn how to create one (Figure 14.2)!

Sometimes when people talk about templates, they're actually referring to slides themselves. And that's OK! Those slides will be based on the template infrastructure, so it makes perfect sense to include slides you use often. We usually refer to these as "starter slides", or "boilerplate slides", or even just "example slides", and most of the templates we create do have some.

OKAY, THEN WHAT IS A THEME?

You may have heard the term "theme" at some point. Don't let that confuse you! A theme is just a variation of a PowerPoint template that doesn't have any slides; it includes only the theme fonts, the theme colours, and the slide layouts. The file extension is .thmx, and if you really want to create a theme, you can open your template and choose Save Current Theme from the bottom of the Themes gallery on the Design tab.

The purpose of a theme is to make it easy for you to apply the same colours and fonts you're using in PowerPoint to your Excel and Word files. To do that, go to the Page Layout tab in Excel or the Design tab in Word, click Themes, and choose a theme there.

When you create your theme you must save it in the folder that opens when you choose Save Current Theme; otherwise, Word and Excel won't see your custom theme (Figure 14.3).

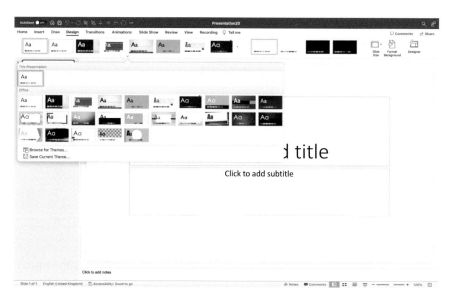

Figure 14.3 The Mac themes gallery.

In PowerPoint, we don't usually recommend applying a theme from the themes gallery to an existing presentation. There are a few reasons for this, but the main one is that it's easy to apply a theme that's not designed for the size of your slide, which will cause the background graphics to become distorted. For example, if you're working with a presentation that uses a 4:3 aspect ratio and you apply a 16:9 theme, any logos included on your master slide and layouts will be squashed. It's usually safer to start a new presentation based on your template or theme and paste in your slides.

THEME VARIANTS

Many of the stock Microsoft themes include what are known as "variants". These enable you to quickly "reskin" the included layouts with new colours and fonts. On the ribbon to the right of the Themes gallery, you will see four (or more!) different choices for your template. Click on these to see the effect on your slides. Just be sure to do this before you customise your template; otherwise, your hard work will be wiped out!

CUSTOMISING A TEMPLATE

You can start with a new, blank file and create your own template completely from scratch. But an easier way to do it is to start with a template you like and customise it to your tastes. For this, we recommend beginning with one of the Microsoft templates.

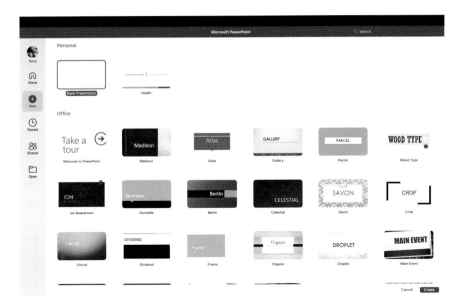

Figure 14.4 Templates Gallery in Backstage View. To get to this screen from Normal View on Mac, select **File** > New from Template. On Windows, choose **File** > New. You can see that we have saved the downloaded Health template and it is now in our Personal options.

We presume you are starting up PowerPoint in Backstage View, as in Figure 14.4. Click **File** > New from Template on Mac or the **File** tab on Windows to open Backstage. Once there, click the New button to open the screen where you can select one of the templates that appear. Or you can search for online templates and themes by typing into the search box. (On Windows, click More Themes and then type in the search box.)

Try typing *Health* there, and then click to download the *Health and fitness* presentation. It might be a good starting point for you. Or *Science* also gives some nice options.

Even if the starter file is labelled as something you won't be presenting on, such as nature, ecology, education, fresh food, or laboratory design, the template infrastructure itself might be perfect for you! And with a few small tweaks, you can make it your own. Of course, you can always start with a new Blank Presentation as well.

SETTING UP THEME FONTS

The first thing you'll want to do to customise your template is to set up the theme fonts. A lot of people skip this step; don't be one of them!

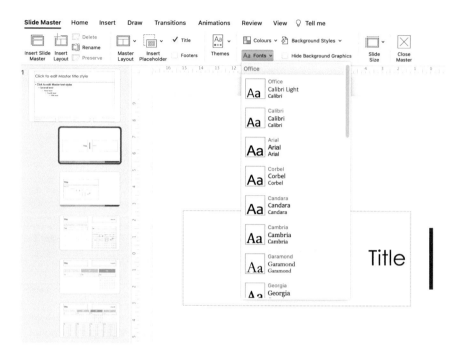

Figure 14.5 The Slide Master tab and the theme font selection. The upper font is the title font and the lower one is the body font.

There are two theme fonts: A heading font and a body font. Slide title placeholders use the theme heading font, and *everything else* uses the theme body font. So that body font is extremely important (Figure 14.5).

The theme body font is used when you create a table, a chart, a text box, a shape or use SmartArt. Similarly, applying a style from the Shape Styles or any other gallery, will also use the theme body font.

A lot of people make the mistake of leaving the theme fonts as-is and applying a font to the placeholders. If you do this the text you type into the placeholders will use the font you applied, but *everything else* will still use the theme font, even if you create it in a placeholder. This causes what we call a Frankendeck, and it will cause you a lot of extra work to format the font on everything to try to make it match. Just let PowerPoint do that work for you!

To choose a different set of theme fonts, open the slide master (**View** > Slide Master), click Fonts, and choose a new set from the menu. The first font listed in each set is the heading font; the second font listed is the body font. They can be the same font.

When you choose the theme font, the heading font will be applied to the title placeholders, and the body font will be applied to all other placeholders.

On the Mac, you're limited to the font sets Microsoft gives you. On Windows, you can create your own set of theme fonts by clicking Customise at the bottom of the Fonts menu in Slide Master View.

If you're working on a Mac and want to create your own set of theme fonts, you'll need to do it in Windows: Open your template file in PowerPoint on Windows, go to Slide Master View, and customise the theme fonts there. Close Slide Master View and save your PowerPoint file. The font theme is now built into the template. Open the file on the Mac and proceed as usual. Of course, you'll want to read the previous chapter on choosing fonts; all of that advice applies here, too!

It's unfortunate that PowerPoint on Mac doesn't let you create customised theme font sets. But here's a little bit of a workaround for you. Choose a theme font set that uses the body font you want for most content. Then, because the header theme font isn't automatically used for anything in PowerPoint other than slide titles, you can apply a non-themed font to the slide title placeholder on the Slide Master. It will then apply that font to the titles on all the slide layouts. At least that can give you a bit more flexibility, although if you update the theme in future, the slide titles will not automatically use the new theme fonts the way the rest of the text will.

SETTING UP THEME COLOURS

Theme colours can be confusing because it's not always obvious what is happening. Just as with the font theme, all content in the file is based on the colour theme by default. When you look at the table, chart, SmartArt, and shape style galleries, you can see that the colour theme is carried throughout all elements and formatting options.

The colour theme is set up with ten theme colours. The first two (labelled A and B in Figure 14.6) are typically used for text colours in tables, SmartArt, shape

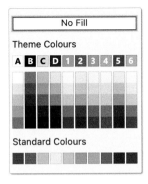

Figure 14.6 PowerPoint's theme colours (with labels added by us).

styles, etc. The second two (labelled C and D) are alternative font and background colours; to be honest, they rarely appear in any of the galleries, although occasionally, Designer in PowerPoint will use them.

The last six colours are called Accent colours—one through six—and appear routinely in all galleries and formatting options. PowerPoint automatically generates a palette of tints and shades based on these ten theme colours.

To customise your theme colours, open Slide Master View (**View** > Slide Master), click Colours, and select from the list of colours. (We like Median a lot.) When you click the colour theme in the list, those colours will be applied to all slide layouts and content, which are now built into the file.

Creating your own colour theme

If you want to create your own colour theme, click Customise Colours at the bottom of the list of theme colour sets (Figure 14.7). You will then see the options in Figure 14.8. Change the colours as desired, give the colour theme a name, and click Save. When you click save, the colours will be applied to all slide layouts and slide content, and they are now built into your file.

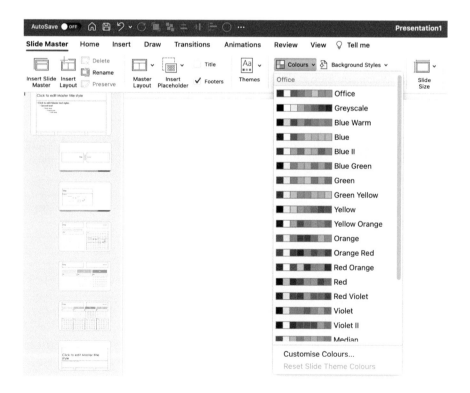

Figure 14.7 The theme colour gallery on a Mac.

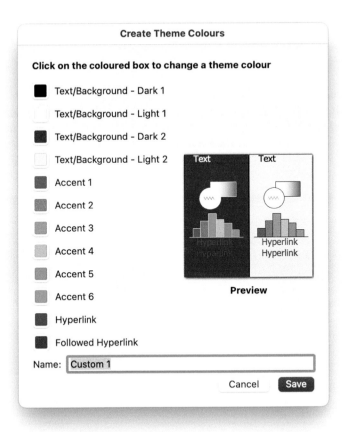

Figure 14.8 Creating new theme colours. It is a good idea to have a clear plan for complementary colours before you start.

Your new colour palette will also be saved in the Colours Gallery under the heading Custom.

Choosing colours that work well together can be challenging, and you may find the Adobe Colour Palette generator or the Coolors website helpful—though these only generate five colour suggestions. These sites provide the hex values for each colour that you can paste into the colour pickers in PowerPoint.

We recommend leaving the first two colours—Text/Background—Dark 1 and Text/Background—Light 1 as black and white. One reason is that you generally want your text to have the most contrast possible, and usually, black and white are your best choices. But also, PowerPoint and Excel will use a tint of Dark 1 as the default font colour in all charts. This isn't anything we can control or change, so if you don't want to start out with bright blue or hot pink chart fonts and have to change them every time, just leave Dark 1 black!

FORMAT THE SLIDE MASTER

Now that you've got your theme fonts and colours set up, you can think about the slide backgrounds.

The slide master is the big thumbnail at the top, and it sets up the basic formatting for **all** the slide layouts. To open the slide master, go to the **View** tab and click Slide Master. Spend a few minutes formatting the placeholders and graphics on the slide master, and then you won't have to repeat it on every layout (Figure 14.9).

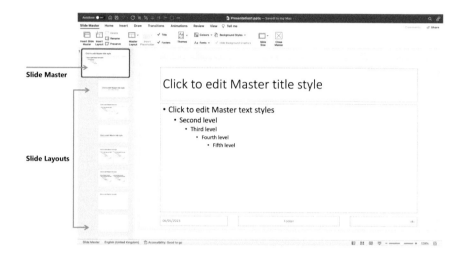

Figure 14.9 Slide master view showing the thumbnails for the slide layouts. The largest thumbnail at the top is the Slide Master. Changes here will affect the individual layouts below.

The first thing is to format and position your slide title. Use the colour, size, and position that you plan to use on the majority of your content slides. Even if you never use any of the content placeholders, the title placeholders keep your slide titles from jumping around as you move from slide to slide—which makes your presentation look much more professional.

Then position and format the font and bullets in the text placeholder. We recommend sticking with a simple round bullet. You want your content to shine, not your choice in bullet points! These settings will automatically apply to all the content placeholders, but you can override them on the individual layouts if you wish.

If any graphical elements, such as a rule line or frame, should appear on most of the content slides, add them to the slide master. We don't recommend adding a

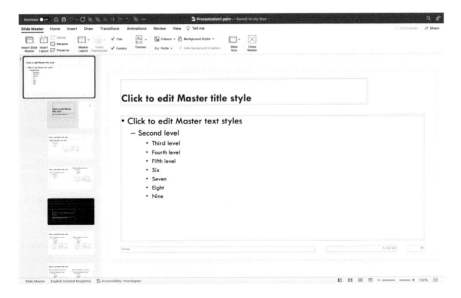

Figure 14.10 **A slide master with various formatting applied.**

logo to every slide, but if you're required to do so, the slide master is where to add it. Just make sure it's small and out of the way because you don't want your content to overlap your logo. Frankly, it looks sloppy, and besides, it breaks all brand guides everywhere (Figure 14.10)!

FORMAT A DARK TITLE SLIDE LAYOUT USING BACKGROUND STYLES

Once you have the basics of the template formatting added to the slide master, it's time to turn your attention to the Title Slide layout. The title slide should stand out from typical content slides, so logos are generally larger than they would be on content slides and the presentation title text is larger and more dramatic.

You may want to make the title slide layout dark to add some drama. It's tempting to change the background colour of the layout, but don't do that! Instead, select the Title Slide layout, and on the Slide Master tab of the Ribbon, click Background Styles and choose one of the dark background styles. Even if it's not the colour you want, that's OK—we'll fix it in a minute.

Changing the background style to a dark colour forces the font colour to change to a light colour. This may not seem important on a title slide because changing the font colour in the two placeholders is easy enough. But it's good to get into the habit of using Background Styles because if you don't when you add charts, SmartArt diagrams, and tables, some of the text might disappear even when it's in a placeholder.

Once you've applied a background style to force the text colour to behave, you can override it with the colour of your choice: right-click in an empty area on the layout or in the pasteboard and select Format Background, then change the background colour in the Format pane. Don't tick Apply to All at the bottom of the Format pane; otherwise you'll mess up all your other layouts.

While you're here, tick the box to Hide Background graphics, which will, as expected, hide the background graphics that were inherited from the slide master.

Now you can use **Insert** > Picture to add your logo to the title slide layout, then size and position it, the text placeholders, and any other graphical elements as desired. Be sure to leave a little breathing room around the edges of the logo. Also, if your logo has a white background, be sure to add a white rectangle to the layout and place your logo on it. If you are adding multiple logos or crests, be sure to align and space them correctly; see Chapter 9. For more information about adding logos and crests, see Chapter 8 (Figure 14.11).

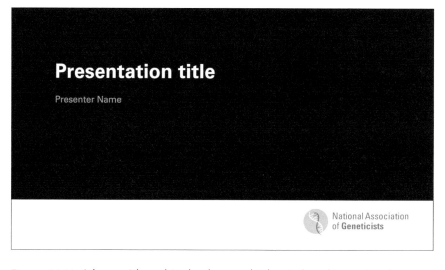

Figure 14.11 A logo with a white background is best placed in a white box or strip.

FORMAT THE REMAINING LAYOUTS

Most stock Microsoft templates have at least a Title Slide layout, a Title and Content layout, a Title Only layout, and a Blank layout with minimal graphics. They may also have layouts such as Two Content, Comparison, Content with Caption, Picture with Caption, etc.

You should be able to use the techniques you learned above to format the remaining layouts by hiding and replacing the graphics inherited from the master or changing the background colour. You can move the placeholders and format the text and bullets appropriately for different uses.

The one thing we'll caution you from doing is adding or deleting placeholders from the layouts that are in the template. If you find that you need to do this, then it's better to create your own custom layout.

CREATE CUSTOM LAYOUTS

There are endless reasons to create custom layouts. Maybe you want to create a variation of a Title Only layout that leaves lots of real estate for charts and tables and omits the logo in the corner, so the content doesn't partially cover it. Or maybe you often have the need for a quotation slide with large text and a picture. Or perhaps you commonly present case studies and need a consistent structure for those. It's really up to you and your imagination!

Creating a custom layout to meet your specific needs (Figure 14.12) is easy. Here are the steps:

1. On the Slide Master tab of the ribbon, choose Insert Layout.
2. Right-click the new layout's thumbnail and choose Rename. Give the layout a short, descriptive name that helps you (and others) remember its intent.
3. Click the arrow beside Insert Placeholder to see the types of placeholders you can add. Choose one, then click and drag on the layout to add it. The Content layout is the most flexible, allowing for text, charts, tables,

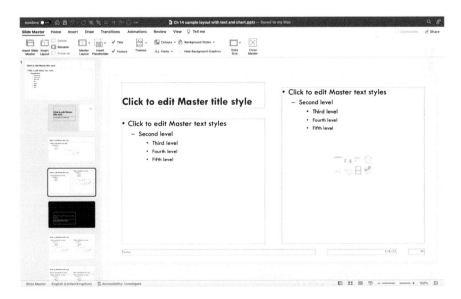

Figure 14.12 A custom layout designed for bulleted explanatory text on the left and content such as charts or SmartArt diagrams on the right.

129

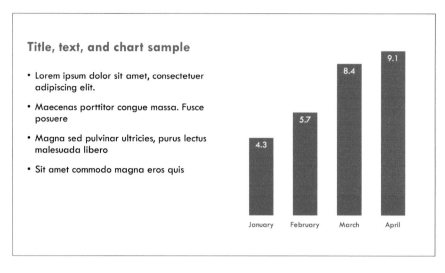

Figure 14.13 An example slide based on the layout in Figure 14.12.

SmartArt, pictures, and other types of content rather than just one specific type of content, such as a chart or a table.

4. Resize and reposition the placeholders as desired.
5. Format text and bullets as needed.

If you don't want to start from scratch, you can right-click an existing slide layout and duplicate it. Rename the duplicate layout and adjust the placeholders to meet your needs.

TEST THE TEMPLATE FILE

After formatting and creating layouts, double-check that they work as you expect. To do so, close Master View, and back in Normal View, click the arrow beside the New Slide button. Select a layout to add a slide based on it.

Insert content into the placeholders to test their functionality. Switch back to Master View and make changes to the layouts as needed. (Be sure you've switched back to Normal View before saving the file.)

Add any boilerplate and starter or often-used slides you want to keep handy.

Now you're ready to save your final template!

SAVE THE TEMPLATE FILE

We started out defining the PowerPoint template as the underlying infrastructure to your file. As you've been working on your template infrastructure, you've probably already saved it a few times. This is a smart thing to do because you don't want to lose your work! When you save the file, by default, it's saved as a PowerPoint Presentation, which has a .pptx extension.

PowerPoint also lets you save the file as a template with a .potx extension. What's the difference? Well, when you double-click a PPTX file in Finder (Mac) or File Explorer (Windows), the operating system opens that presentation file itself. You make changes to it and save those changes. When you double-click a POTX, the operating system opens a new file based on the template and leaves the original template file alone. This way your template file remains intact, and you don't inadvertently mess it up.

You can keep your final "template" file as a PPTX if you want. The template infrastructure is built in, so you don't have to keep it as a POTX.

Even so, you should save your template as a POTX one time before you finalise it. Saving as POTX breaks the file's connection to the stock Microsoft theme variants. These aren't important to you unless you click on one accidentally or if you change the slide size. In those cases, the Microsoft formatting will override your custom setup! If you don't want to lose your hard work, be sure to save your file as a POTX. After that, you can re-save it as a PPTX if you want.

Developing your own templates is great fun and allows you to produce your unique slide styles. We have only scratched the surface here. If you want to dive deeper into this subject, you might want to read our book, Building PowerPoint Templates v2.

PART 3

Showing data

15

Creating tables and charts

Most scientific presentations will, of necessity, contain data. PowerPoint encourages you to show these data as tables or in charts. So what is the difference between a table, a chart and a graph?

A chart is defined as information in the form of a table, graph, or diagram; thus, strictly speaking, "chart" is an over-arching term for all of these. A table is information systematically displayed, most commonly in columns and rows. A graph is an illustration showing the relation between variables measured along one of a pair of axes at right angles. The terms chart and graph are often used interchangeably, as we will do here. PowerPoint uses the term chart in reference to graphs.

Let's imagine that you are sitting at a team briefing. Someone has brought performance data to the meeting, including a printed Excel spreadsheet. Your first instinct is to look at the Excel table, running your finger along the rows and columns to see how you are performing.

If the same data is projected, your eye tries to replicate this action. You find the relevant row and then try to scan across the row, while taking in what the individual columns are. This takes time and it is easy to make mistakes. Meanwhile, you are not listening to what is being said!

Tables are a poor way to communicate complex data, but if there is no alternative, you at least need to format the table so that the audience gets the message immediately. In this chapter we will focus on inserting tables and charts with basic formatting. In the next chapter, we'll talk about some basic principles for more effective data visualisation.

CREATING A TABLE IN PowerPoint

To insert a table, click the Table button on the **Insert** tab and drag over the grid to select the number of rows and columns, or click **Insert** > Table > Insert Table, and tell PowerPoint specifically how many rows and columns you need.

DOI: 10.1201/9781003287902-18

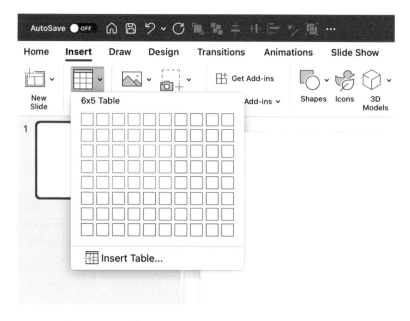

Figure 15.1 The Insert Table graphical interface on a Mac.

PowerPoint will create the table using the file's theme colours, the theme body font, and banded (shaded) rows (Figure 15.1).

Table style formatting

To quickly format the table, select it and choose one of the options from the **Table Design** > Table Styles gallery. These styles are based on the theme colours in your file, and some are easier on the eyes than others!

We generally recommend that you choose one of the options labelled Light Style 1, preferably one with light grey banded rows if possible. If you don't have an option with light grey, opt for light blue or green rather than pink or yellow.

Once you've applied a table style, you can tick the boxes for the various Table Style Options to toggle formatting for the banded rows and columns, the header and total rows, and the first and last columns. It's worth trying these to see if they can save you some manual formatting time! We will cover table style options in more detail in Chapter 16.

Manual formatting

Often, the table styles won't do exactly what you want. In those cases, you'll need to manually format the table.

As with most things in PowerPoint, you must select the object before you can format it. Click and drag over cells to select them. You can also hover just outside a row or column and when your cursor turns into a small arrow, click to select the row or column. On Mac, you can right-click in a cell and choose Select > Select Column or Select Row; on Windows, right-click in a cell and select these from the floating minibar.

Once you've selected the cells you wish to format, choose **Table Design** > Shading to apply a colour fill. For borders, the tools feel a bit backwards on the Ribbon. Start at the far right to change the border formatting by choosing Pen Colour, Pen Weight (thick or thin) and Pen Style (dashed or solid). From there, move to the left, click on Borders and then select from the dropdown to apply the appropriate borders.

Table borders can be fiddly; sometimes, to remove a border, you'll need to apply formatting and then apply it again to actually turn it off! Don't let that throw you—just repeat the Borders > Border selection to toggle the formatting on and off. We tend to select all the cells in the table, apply inside horizontal borders, and turn off the outside borders for a cleaner look.

Inserting tables from Excel

Sometimes you may need to insert spreadsheet cells or tables from Excel. Select and copy the cells in Excel, then paste the table onto the slide using Ctrl [⌘] + V. Immediately click the Paste Options button to see your choices.

On Mac, you'll see a list of options. On Windows, it's a set of icons; hover over them to help identify what's what.

Use Destination Theme is the default paste option (shown in Figure 15.2). This pastes your Excel content as a PowerPoint table and applies basic formatting

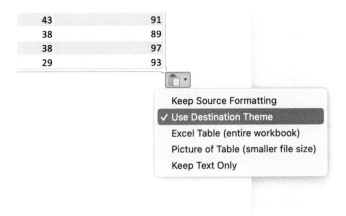

Figure 15.2 After pasting a table from Excel, the options are shown in a drop-down menu.

based on your PowerPoint theme. Use the formatting techniques described above to format the table.

Keep Source Formatting also pastes your content as a PowerPoint table, but it keeps the formatting you applied in Excel.

Excel Table (entire workbook) embeds the Excel workbook into your presentation. You'll need to use this option if you've added conditional formatting, data bars, or sparklines (or other similar features that PowerPoint tables don't have) that you want to show in your table in PowerPoint. Remember, this embeds the entire Excel workbook, not just the single worksheet.

Picture of Table (smaller file size) inserts a picture of the table. This means the table and data won't be editable on the slide, and if you need to resize the picture, be sure to press Shift and drag from a corner so the text isn't distorted.

Keep Text Only pastes all the text from the table into a text box with tabs separating the text.

Starting a chart in PowerPoint

Charts are the mainstay of data presentation. There are two main ways to get charts into PowerPoint slides: start in PowerPoint or start in Excel. Our preferred method is to start the process in PowerPoint.

Often users insert a new slide and choose Title and Content from **Home** > New Slide, then click on the chart icon in the placeholder and select the chart type. Depending on your template, this sometimes gives you a slide with a title and a chart where the chart fills only about one-third of the slide area.

Charts are much easier to interpret if they fill most of the slide, so in that case, create a Title Only slide and select **Insert** > Chart.

The Insert Chart galleries look a little different in Mac and Windows, but the same charts are included in both. A clustered column chart is the most common chart used in medical presentations, and you usually won't go wrong choosing a 2D clustered column or bar.

Once you choose a chart type and insert the chart, an example chart is created, and an Excel spreadsheet opens. On Mac, you will see the Excel ribbon tools; on Windows, click the button in the data sheet that's labelled Edit Data in Microsoft Excel if you need to access the full Excel tools for sorting and adding formulas, etc. In both, you'll know the chart is included in the PowerPoint file and not a separate Excel file because it will say *Chart in Microsoft PowerPoint* at the top of the datasheet.

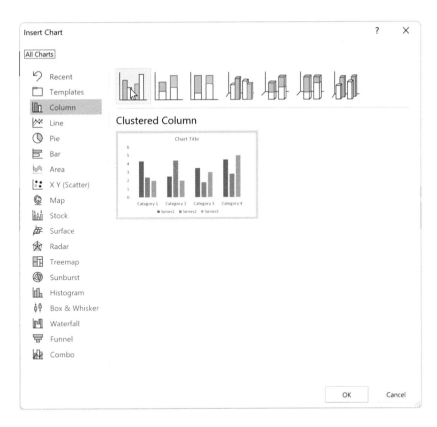

Figure 15.3 Selecting your preferred chart type on Windows.

When you start your chart from PowerPoint, the datasheet is pre-populated with dummy data that you can replace with your own. If you're unsure how the data should be entered to create a specific type of chart in Excel, the example data PowerPoint provides is a useful guide (Figures 15.3 and 15.4).

If you already have data in Excel, simply open that workbook and copy only the data you need. Then paste this into the Excel data sheet that PowerPoint has opened. A little blue outline around your data shows which cells PowerPoint uses for the chart. If your chart seems to be missing some data, check that this blue outline is correctly placed (Figure 15.5).

Categories will be shown along the horizontal axis when you create a column or line chart in PowerPoint by default. If you'd prefer that the data series be shown there instead, you don't have to change the data in the spreadsheet. Instead, choose Switch Row and Column on the **Chart Design** tab to swap the categories and series in the chart.

You can also sort the data in Excel, either from highest to lowest or vice versa.

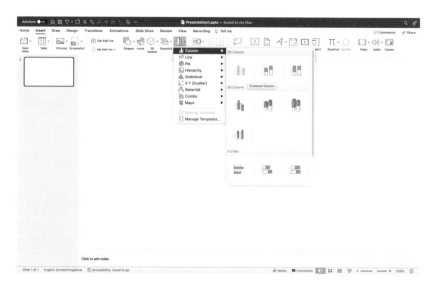

Figure 15.4 Inserting the same chart on a Mac.

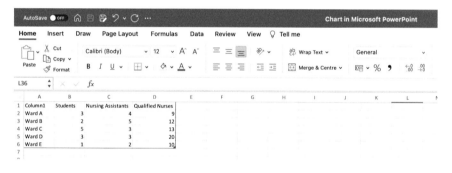

Figure 15.5 The data selection in Excel. The blue box outlines the data to be included in the chart.

When you are satisfied with the basic chart data, you can close the spreadsheet. If you need to open it again, right-click the chart and choose Edit Data (Windows) or Edit Data in Excel (Mac).

Starting a chart in Excel

You may already have data in a spreadsheet and prefer to create the chart in Excel proper. In that case, you can copy the chart and paste it into your slide. Immediately after you paste the chart, a small paste options icon will appear beside it. Click on this before you do anything else. You can choose between linking the data, embedding the workbook, or pasting a picture of the chart. It is important that you understand the difference (Figures 15.6 and 15.7).

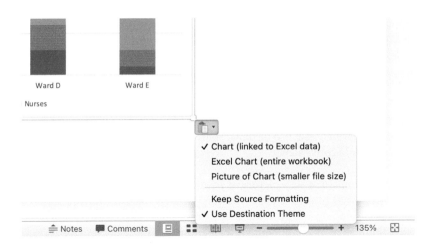

Figure 15.6 The options when pasting an Excel chart into PowerPoint on a Mac.

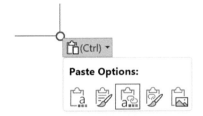

Figure 15.7 The options when pasting an Excel chart into PowerPoint in Windows; hover over each paste option icon to see its behaviour.

Linking to Excel data creates a connection between the chart in the PowerPoint file and the Excel spreadsheet. Rather than dumping all of the data from the workbook into your presentation, it's maintained in the original Excel file. You'll still be able to format the chart, but if you want to edit the actual data, you'll need access to the Excel workbook.

With linked data, when you email the presentation to someone else, they cannot update the data in the chart unless they have access to the Excel workbook. But that also means that you will want to have access to your Excel file so you can update it if you need to! An easy way to ensure that the links work for you is to put the Excel and PowerPoint files into the same folder before copying and pasting your chart from Excel onto your slide.

Do note that if you use Ctrl + V (Windows) or ⌘ + V (Mac) to paste the chart, you'll get linked data by default. Of course, you can change this with the Paste Options icon, which is why we pointed it out!

Conversely, embedding the chart will transfer *all* the information from your Excel workbook into the PowerPoint file. This may produce a very large presentation file, so be careful. Most importantly, anyone with access to the PowerPoint file can also access *the entire Excel file*. There may be information such as confidential patient or institutional data in the workbook, even if it's not on the specific spreadsheet your chart is on. Sometimes embedding an Excel workbook is tempting because all the information is right there, self-contained in the PowerPoint file; but it can also be dangerous, so don't get yourself into trouble for the sake of a little convenience.

The final option is to paste a picture of your chart, but you will be unable to edit the chart in PowerPoint. Of course, you can always go back to Excel to make edits and repeat the copy-paste process. This is certainly a very safe option if you are worried about sharing confidential information.

Formatting your chart

The formatting options for charts are a bit different depending if you're working on a Mac or a Windows system.

In Windows, selecting the chart enables a set of "charms", allowing you to quickly enable or disable various chart elements such as axes, labels, and gridlines. Choosing More Options from the flyout opens the Format Pane, which gives you access to additional settings.

In the Mac interface, you'll use the formatting tools on the contextual **Format** tab (which is also available in Windows), and you can open the Format Task Pane from here as well (which you cannot do in Windows). Mac PowerPoint doesn't add charms to the chart, but you can turn elements on and off on the contextual **Chart Design** tab under Add Chart Element. Finally, in both Mac and Windows, you can always right-click on a chart element and choose Format <element> to open the Format Pane (Figures 15.8 and 15.9).

You may not need a chart title; we often see slides with an identical slide and chart title. You may choose to include a "call to action" or key takeaway rather than a title. To get rid of the chart title, click to select the title text box and disable it using the Add Chart Elements menu (Mac) or the charms (Windows), or simply delete it by hitting the Delete key on your keyboard.

We often remove the major gridlines on the vertical axis as well. To do so, click carefully on one of the light horizontal lines to select them, then disable or delete them as you would with the chart title.

The colour of each chart element is defined by your theme colours. In Chapter 14 we showed you how to change these. You may prefer to change the theme colours overall or manually change the formatting of the individual chart elements. It

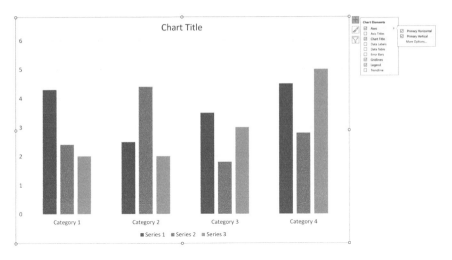

Figure 15.8 On Windows, charms let you enable various chart elements.

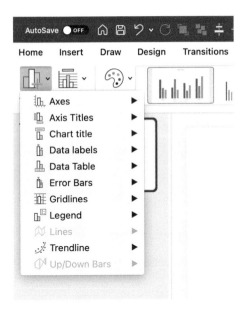

Figure 15.9 On Mac, use **Chart Design** > Add Chart Element to enable various Chart Elements.

can be better to change the default colour theme so that all your charts use the same scheme by default but be careful when updating theme colours because this will affect everything in your file, which may be more trouble than it's worth.

Clicking once on any column will select all the columns in that category or series; clicking a second time will select only that single column. (Clicking a second time is how you select an individual data point or data label in all charts, not just column charts.) You can then use the Shape Fill option on the **Home** tab, the contextual **Format** tab, or the Format pane to select a different colour.

You can also alter the width of the data series columns and the gap between them. Click on any data column in the chart. Then open the Format Pane if it's not already visible. (Use **Format** > Format Pane on Mac or right-click > Format Data Series on Windows.) Adjust the Series Overlap and Gap Width sliders in the Format Pane under Series Options (the chart icon). You want the columns to be reasonably thick, with a small gap between series and a larger gap between categories.

You can also change the appearance of the axes. Right-click on an axis and select Format Axis to open the Format Pane to the Axis Options tab. It is worth trying different settings on the Axis Options tab to see how they affect the axes. Adjust minimum and maximum in the Format Pane > Axis Options (the chart icon), change the line colour and thickness under Fill & Line (the paint bucket icon), and change the size and colour of the axis text on the **Home** tab of the Ribbon (Figure 15.10).

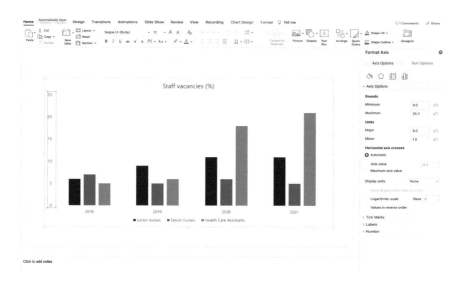

Figure 15.10 Adjust the Axis settings on the Axis Options tab of the Format Pane.

Quick chart formatting options

PowerPoint does give you quite a few options for one-click formatting on the Chart Design tab. We're not fond of the chart styles, but the Quick Layout options are great! We especially like Layout 2 because it adds data labels and removes the redundant axis with one click. Even if it's not exactly what we ultimately want, it often gets us at least 90% of the way there.

Be sure to check out the Change Colours dropdown also. The options here offer a fast way to apply a monochromatic scale of colours to your charts, so you don't have to waste time selecting specific colours from the theme colour palette.

Chart templates

Once you have formatted a chart exactly as you wish, you can save that formatting as a template for future use. Right-click on the chart and choose Save As Template. Give the template a unique name. Do not change where PowerPoint wants to save it so that when you are ready to use the chart template, the software can find it again.

You may want to create a chart with extra data series and format those before saving the chart template; that way, your chart template can be easily used on charts with lots of series. Be especially mindful of the axis settings because they will be included with your chart template. For example, if you've created a chart template that uses currency on the value axis, applying this template to another chart will change its axis to use currency as well.

Once you have inserted a new chart, you can change the appearance to the saved chart template by right-clicking on the chart and selecting **Chart Design** > Change Chart Type > Templates > Your Chart Template (Figure 15.11).

Even better, when you want to insert a new chart, either in this presentation or one in the future, you can insert it using your customised chart template; select **Insert** > Chart > Templates > Your Chart Template.

Changing chart types

You can change the chart type using the **Insert** > Chart menu. For example, you may have a pie chart you want to change to a column chart. Select your existing pie chart, then go to **Insert** > Chart and from the drop-down menu (Mac) or dialogue (Windows), choose Column > Clustered Column.

You can also select the chart and use **Chart Design** > Change Chart Type, then choose a different chart.

Common chart types

There are a huge number of different chart types, so how do you choose the correct one? In reality, only a limited range of chart types are necessary. It may also be that a simple number placed front and centre on your slide with a brief explanatory statement is enough, and you don't need a chart at all.

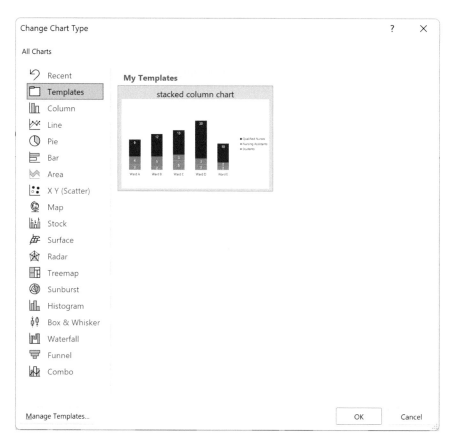

Figure 15.11 Using a chart template to change the appearance of a chart to a custom design in Windows. The options are the same on a Mac.

BAR CHARTS

Bar charts are probably the most common chart used in medical presentations. There may be more than one series in a category or more than one category in a series. You'll rarely go wrong with a bar chart; however, you should avoid putting too much data in any one chart.

We often see vertical bar charts, called column charts in PowerPoint, where long labels on the axis are either abbreviated or lie diagonally, which is difficult to read. This is a sure sign that the vertical bar chart needs to be changed to a horizontal bar chart, where the bars run horizontally rather than vertically—duh! Horizontal bar charts are one of the easiest charts to read.

Stacked vertical bar charts are a sub-category where the data in each column is broken down for comparison. For example, each vertical bar in a chart comparing

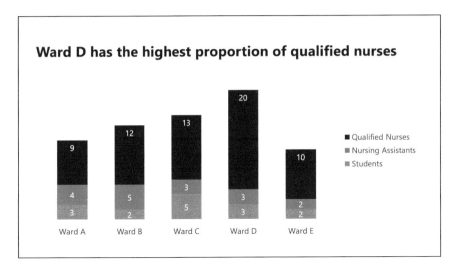

Figure 15.12 **A stacked column chart.**

wards with each other may be subdivided by the number of student nurses, qualified nurses and nursing assistants. These will be colour-coded within each stacked bar (Figure 15.12).

PIE CHARTS

Pie charts are grossly overused (and overvalued). Ironically, the icon for PowerPoint in Microsoft 365 is a pie chart; this is possibly the least useful visual for conveying comparative data! There has been much speculation about how they are interpreted. It seems likely that the length of the arc is what the human eye tries to assess rather than the area of the slice.

Pie charts are useful when you are trying to show parts of a whole and when there are only a limited number of variables. Say, for example, you have three possible responses to a question: Yes, No, or Undecided. A pie chart could be used here.

If there are too many variables, pie charts are hard to read. Similarly, a pie chart is not the best solution if the data shows very similar amounts for each category.

When using a pie chart, keep it clean and simple. Never use 3D, as the distortion makes interpretation even harder, and don't explode segments of the chart. (Remember, the viewer is trying to estimate the length of the arc.) Best practices recommend keeping the number of slices to five or fewer.

Donut charts are a variant of pie charts with a hole in the middle. They suffer the same limitations in data interpretation as pies. Donuts are great, donut charts less so.

If you find yourself needing too many slices of pies and donuts (see what we did there?), consider using a column or bar chart, a stacked column or bar, a treemap, or perhaps a waffle chart instead. Columns and bars, stacked columns and bars, and slope charts are good alternatives to using multiple pies for comparison.

SCATTERPLOTS

Scatterplots show the relationship between two data sets, such as the number of nursing staff on duty relating to the number of falls per month on a ward (Figure 15.13). (These are fictitious data.)

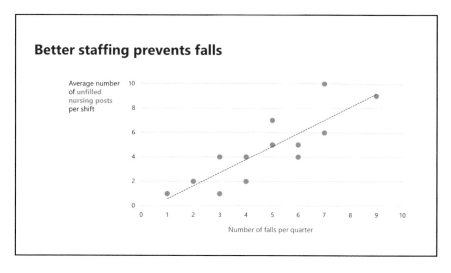

Figure 15.13 A scatterplot showing the data on falls relating to staffing levels, with a trend line included.

LINE CHARTS

Line charts are typically used to show changes over time, where time is plotted on the X axis, for example, when looking at medication costs by year. Line charts are also especially useful to show the overall shape of the data, which is good for highlighting trends (Figure 15.14).

WATERFALL CHART

A waterfall chart can be used if data may vary either side of a baseline, typically for financial data. A waterfall chart could be used to examine staff turnover, where newly appointed staff raise the bars vertically and staff leaving cause it to fall below the baseline (Figure 15.15).

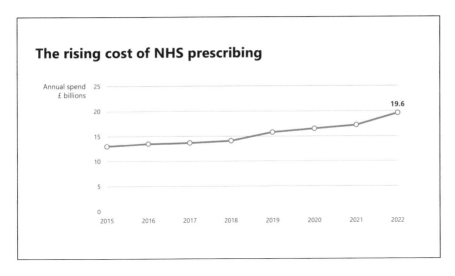

Figure 15.14 The rising cost of NHS spending shown as a line graph.

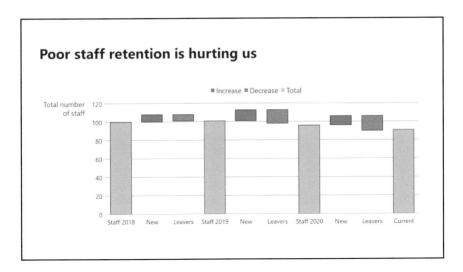

Figure 15.15 A waterfall chart used to show staff turnover.

SLOPE CHARTS

Slope charts are very underused. They are great for showing changes between two variables, whether it's two years, men vs women, or kids vs adults. The change before and after an intervention or a time interval can be visualised in a slope chart.

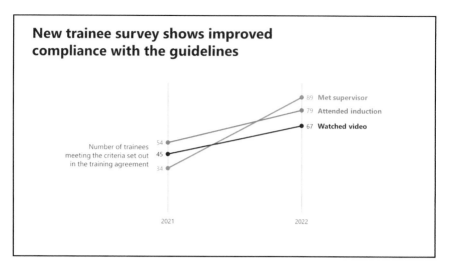

New trainee survey shows improved compliance with the guidelines

Figure 15.16 A slope chart showing trainee compliance with guidelines improving between two data collection points.

For example Figure 15.16 shows the results of an annual survey of new trainees, assessing their compliance with local policy.

Conclusion

Tables and charts are a great way to display data in presentations. However, it is important to give careful thought to which chart is best for your data. Try to keep chart and chart styles consistent throughout your slide deck.

Think about whether your chosen chart allows the viewer to understand your message at a glance. If not, be sure to read Chapter 16, which will help you understand the basics of data visualisation and get your point across more effectively.

16

Data visualisation

Data visualisation and storytelling are popular terms these days. They sound complex and time-consuming, but don't let them fool you. All those terms really mean is, what am I trying to say with this slide, and is it understandable at a glance? If not, then you need to rethink your design.

In earlier chapters, we talked about less is more, but nowhere is this more important than when you're displaying data. It's pointless to dump a spreadsheet onto a slide and expect your audience to figure out what's important. You're not in school; you don't have to show your work. Sure, you can keep those spreadsheets in your back pocket in case someone wants to see all the data but don't expect them to do the hard work of explaining the salient points. That is your job.

If we refer to the beginning of the book where we discussed cognitive load, it's a good reminder that we need to apply these principles to our chart and table designs as well as to the overall slide designs. Think of your slides as billboards; the reader should be able to understand the primary information *at a glance*. Extra information and visual clutter contribute to cognitive overload, which often obscures the point we're trying to make. The lesson here is to keep your charts and table clean and highlight what's important for your audience to understand.

How do we do this? It's really not difficult. You just have to know what you're trying to say (which we admit is sometimes the hardest part!) and take the time to make sure that information stands out.

Leveraging pre-attentive attributes can help with that.

PRE-ATTENTIVE ATTRIBUTES

Pre-attentive attributes are the visual things our brains start noticing and sorting through before we even realise it. It's the stuff we notice subconsciously when we're looking at visual information—which includes charts and tables.

Adding emphasis, contrast, and white space will help call out specific data, which helps your audience know what to focus on and subconsciously begin to interpret the information before you even begin speaking.

If you understand these things you can make better design decisions. Tapping into pre-attentive processing will help you make specific information stand out.

Creating emphasis

Creating emphasis is mostly about creating contrast. Contrast identifies the important information on your slide. Your eye will naturally look at the area of most contrast. It's one of the easiest ways to add visual interest to your charts and makes your audience want to look at the information you are presenting. It also tells your audience exactly what they should be paying attention to before they're even consciously paying attention!

Colour and size are two of the most effective ways to create contrast on slides and in charts because they establish a hierarchy of information. The important thing to remember is that for contrast to be effective, it has to be strong, and it has to be bold.

Getting rid of chart junk

Chart junk is a term coined by Edward Tufte in 1983, and it refers to any visual element in a chart that is distracting or doesn't help you understand the data. Chart junk can include unnecessary gridlines, redundant axis and data labels, 3D formatting, numbers with lots of extra zeros (1,000,000 vs 1M, for example) and decimal places, etc.

An element that might be necessary on one chart could be considered junk on another. Part of your job as a chart designer is to consider all the elements on each chart, determine if any of them contribute to visual clutter, and see if you can remove them.

White space is non-negotiable

You must have white space in order to create contrast and emphasis.

White space doesn't have to be white—it just has to be empty. You'll sometimes hear it called negative space. As with contrast, white space helps identify the key information in your chart. It calls attention to the important bits and gives your eye a place to rest.

We often see charts where every line is super thick and all different colours and styles and all the text is bold, and every gridline and axis label is black. The chart designer has piled on more and more colour and more and more boldness in an effort to make things stand out. But honestly, the result is that we simply have no idea where to look. Remember, when everything is bold, nothing is bold. It's your job to determine what's important. Make that thing bold and then tone back everything else.

Don't be afraid of white space. By stripping off all the chart junk and by emphasising the important bits, your audience members automatically know what's important and they know where to look. And by making it easier for your audience to focus on your data, you make it easier for yourself to make your points more effectively.

Let's look at some examples using fictitious data.

STARTING WITH A TABLE

Our data story is as follows. The British Society of Gastroenterology recommends that endoscopists should have a caecal intubation rate of at least 90%. We have conducted a review of self-reported colonoscopy data from 12 endoscopists in four local hospitals.

After a little time going through the data, we can see that five endoscopists do not meet this target. We want to articulate this (diplomatically) and make some recommendations for change.

This is what the default table will look like when added to a PowerPoint slide (Figure 16.1).

Site	Colonoscopist	Mean sedation	Number of cases	Adenoma detection rate	Caecal intubation rate
Hospital A	A	2.75	145	25	92
Hospital A	B	3.25	187	26	84
Hospital A	C	3.12	220	34	89
Hospital B	D	3.41	320	28	88
Hospital B	E	1.89	301	34	93
Hospital B	F	2.56	322	43	95
Hospital C	G	4.82	87	17	76
Hospital C	H	2.6	289	45	92
Hospital D	I	1.98	290	43	91
Hospital D	J	1.99	360	38	89
Hospital D	K	2.2	198	38	97
Hospital D	L	2.71	258	29	93

Figure 16.1 PowerPoint's default table.

The extra colour and banded rows don't help us understand what's important. Cutting down on this type of "table junk" can make the table easier to understand.

Getting rid of table junk

Remember, the goal here is to get rid of unnecessary gridlines and shading that clutter the table and obscure the information. If you prefer to just choose one of PowerPoint's table styles, open the Table Styles gallery from the **Table Design** tab and choose one of the simpler table styles. We like Light Style 1 because it has simple shaded rows and few extra gridlines. If you prefer one of the other styles you can always use it as a starting point, then remove gridlines or turn off the banded rows as needed. But do take the time to clean up your tables because the default PowerPoint table style is, frankly, not very helpful for reading and understanding the data within (Figure 16.2).

Start by stripping the table of all gridlines. You can then add back internal horizontal gridlines to help the readers' eye move across the line more easily. Just be sure to use light gridlines—you'll never go wrong with a light grey—otherwise, all your data will be hard to see in the sea of black lines!

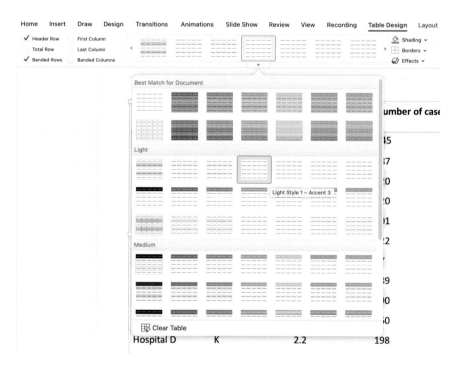

Figure 16.2 The table styles gallery, with LightStyle 1 – Accent 3 applied.

Also, you usually don't need both gridlines and filled (banded) rows like you often get with the PowerPoint table styles. Choose one or the other. For fills, choose the lightest grey for one row and then no fill for the next.

Add contrast to the data you want to highlight. In Figure 16.3, we added shading to emphasise the five colonoscopists below the desired 90% threshold, and we added that key takeaway to the slide title as well. Even without a lot of colour, it's clear that these are the data points we should focus on.

Over **40%** of endoscopists miss the BSG target of a **90%** caecal intubation rate	Colonoscopist	Mean sedation	Number of cases	Adenoma detection rate	Caecal intubation rate
	A	2.75	145	25	92
	B	3.25	187	26	84
	C	3.12	220	34	89
	D	3.41	320	28	88
	E	1.89	301	34	93
	F	2.56	322	43	95
	G	4.82	87	17	76
	H	2.6	289	45	92
	I	1.98	290	43	91
	J	1.99	360	38	89
	K	2.2	198	38	97
	L	2.71	258	29	93

Figure 16.3 Cleaned-up table emphasising the data the audience should focus on.

It is worth stating that it is unlikely that you would want to name and shame your colleagues, so the data in the original table has been anonymised—or has it? If you work with this group, you will know that Hospital C is the only one with two endoscopists, one of whom does many more procedures than the other. Be very careful with data that you think might be anonymous but isn't. For this reason, we've removed the identifying hospital column from the final table.

Short bits of text can often be centred, as you see in the first column of Figure 16.3, but text is almost always easier to read when left-aligned. The number columns are right-aligned to help with readability. Although you can add decimal tabs to columns in PowerPoint, it's tedious to do so. In this case, we used a little hack: We just added zeroes where necessary to force the correct alignment and then coloured them the same as the cell fill so they don't show.

One final tweak: No one measures sedation in tenths of a mg. Just round those numbers up or down!

IMPROVING A BASIC COLUMN CHART

The cleaned-up table above is fine, but it might be easier for the audience to understand the important information if we create a column chart instead (Figure 16.4).

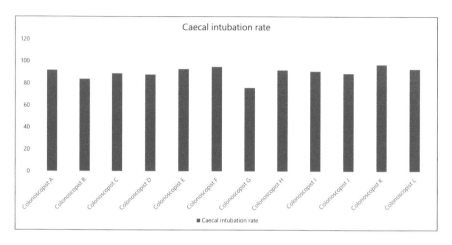

Figure 16.4 PowerPoint's default column chart.

You'll rarely go wrong with a column chart, but you can definitely make some improvements. You don't need both the axis labels and the data labels—or even a legend—in this simple chart.

When you see the labels on the x-axis are at an angle, you need to fix them. No one wants to angle their head to read your chart! In most cases, the solution is to change the chart type to a horizontal bar chart. The labels will now run across the slide.

However in this case, you can remove the redundant "colonoscopist" text from each data point and add that to the chart or slide title. In addition to cutting down on clutter, the axis text is no longer presented at an angle, which makes it infinitely easier to read.

Making the bars wider is usually more visually pleasing, enabling us to add a data label to the inside end of each bar. (Data labels can go inside the bars or outside, or even a mix of the two when needed.) Adding data labels enables us to remove the now-redundant value axis labels.

You also don't need to make every bar a different colour. In fact keeping all the bars the same colour reduces cognitive load and encourages us to compare the data as a whole. If you add a lot of colour to a simple chart like this, the audience

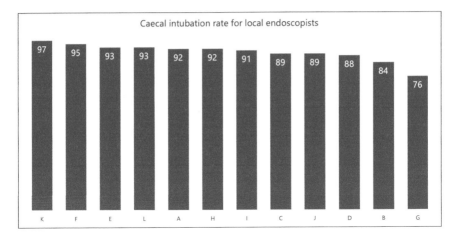

Figure 16.5 **Column chart with some tweaks.**

will wonder if the different colours have meaning rather than focusing on what you have to say. Too much colour also makes it difficult to make your focal point stand out.

Sorting data often makes it easier to parse the information at a glance. (Sorting data can be helpful in tables also, but PowerPoint tables unfortunately don't have any sorting tools.) We ranked the endoscopists in our example from highest to lowest intubation rate by sorting the data points in the chart data sheet (Figure 16.5).

Finally, you should be aware that the value axis for bar charts, whether horizontal or vertical, should always begin at zero. This is because of pre-attentive attributes; our brains interpret the length of the bar from the baseline axis as we're assessing the overall data. Therefore, to have a bar begin at a number other than zero is visually misleading. If you need a shorter axis so you can see tiny differences in the data or if the evaluation scale doesn't start at zero (pH, for example), consider using a line chart instead. Other charts to consider include a dot plot, a dumbbell or lollipop, a bee swarm, or various other types of charts. Check sources like storytellingwithdata.com or evergreendata.com for inspiration.

Telling the story of the data

That is certainly a clearer chart, but what story are we trying to tell? To take our example a step further, we've changed the title to a descriptive headline, so the audience immediately understands the chart. We've also added contrast to the data bars. This uses pre-attentive attributes to draw the viewer's eye to the key message and reinforce the headline. Now it's much easier to pick up on the fact that five of the endoscopists aren't meeting that 90% goal (Figure 16.6).

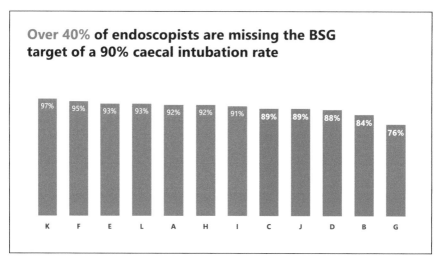

Figure 16.6 This chart and headline reinforce the message of the data.

USING DIRECT OR "IN-LINE" LABELS

Whenever possible, it's better to label data points directly rather than using a legend. This prevents your audience from bouncing back and forth between the data and the legend, lessening cognitive load and making the chart easier to understand. When column charts have multiple data series, it's often difficult to do, and in those cases, definitely keep the legend intact, as you can see in Figure 16.7.

As a general rule, data showing change over time is best displayed as a line chart because trends and the shape of the data are more obvious. The added bonus here

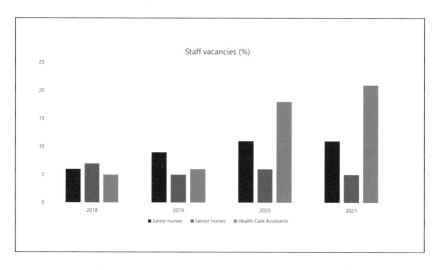

Figure 16.7 A column chart showing vacancies by year and staff type.

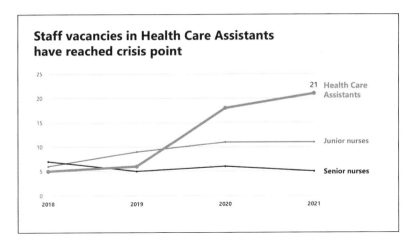

Staff vacancies in Health Care Assistants have reached crisis point

Figure 16.8 A line chart showing changes in the data over time.

is that line charts are usually easy to label directly rather than relying on a legend. This also means you don't have to use weird dashes and colours to distinguish one line from another (Figure 16.8).

It should be obvious that we've tapped into some pre-attentive attributes to make this line chart quicker to read at a glance by removing all chart junk and adding colour and weight to the data we want to focus on.

STATEMENT SLIDES

Remember also that you don't always need a chart. Sometimes a simple statement slide is enough (Figure 16.9).

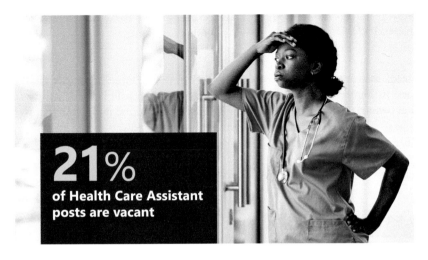

Figure 16.9 A simple statement is a great way to get your message across.

TOO MUCH PIE IS BAD FOR YOU

Presenters love pie charts. But it's worth remembering that just because it adds up to 100% doesn't mean it has to be a pie.

Most importantly, as we stated in Chapter 15, if there are more than five slices in your pie, you should try to find a better way to display the data. Figure 16.10 should be an obvious example of too many slices in a pie, but apparently, it's not obvious enough because we see these frequently! Even changing the legend to direct labels and adding a highlight colour to help with pre-attentive processing cannot be effective with a chart like this.

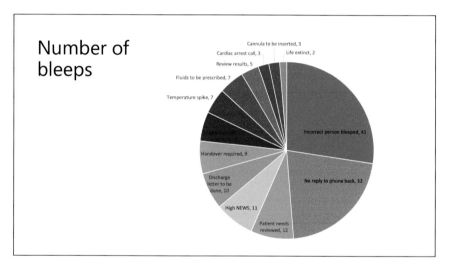

Figure 16.10 This default pie chart has too many slices to be effective. (Slide provided by Dr Gareth Lewis.)

Instead, convert that pie into a chart where you can actually see the data. As shown in Figure 16.11, a bar chart is almost always a safe bet, with the additional benefit that long data labels can be easily accommodated. Note that we've emphasised the relevant data and placed the key takeaway in the slide title as well.

Figure 16.12 shows a treemap with the same data. A treemap can be a good alternative to a crowded pie chart.

MAPS

Maps are available as a chart type in PowerPoint. You can add a true map chart using **Insert** > Chart > Maps. As with any other chart, PowerPoint will open a

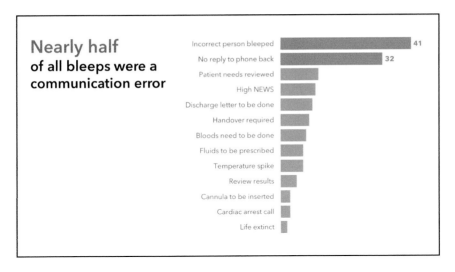

Figure 16.11 Long data labels are begging for a horizontal bar chart. (Slide provided by Dr Gareth Lewis.)

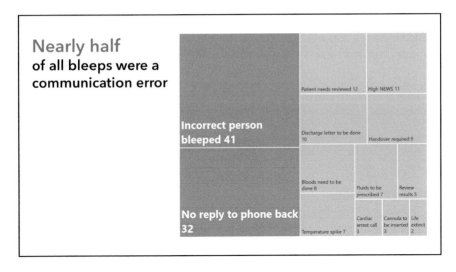

Figure 16.12 Using colour and contrast draws the eye to the take-home message in this treemap.

spreadsheet with dummy data that you can edit, and the map will adjust. You can then change the colours of individual data sets (countries) just as in a chart!

You can also add vector map graphics to your slide and manually recolour the geographic areas as needed Figure 16.13. You can find vector maps on various sites, such as istockphoto.com and freevectormaps.com.

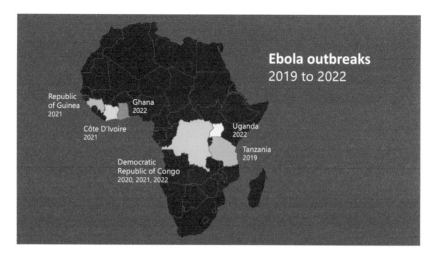

Figure 16.13 Example of a vector map which has been recoloured to highlight specific data.

ICON ARRAYS

Let's imagine your research shows that only 47% of businesses have readily available defibrillators. A simple statistic like this can be nicely represented with an icon array, which (as you might imagine from the name) uses icons to represent the data.

Insert your icon, duplicate it, align it, and space it evenly to create a row of 10. Then duplicate that row to complete your grid of 100 icons, each representing 1 percent. Colour as many icons as necessary to represent your data, as shown in Figure 16.14.

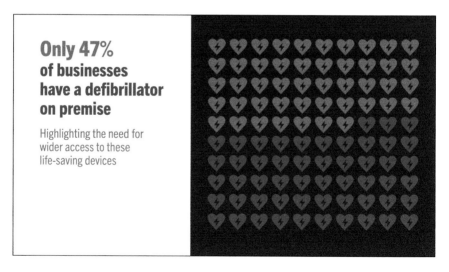

Figure 16.14 Using icons to represent data can bring a different look to your slides.

Don't try to split or colour half of an icon! If you're talking about 46.5%, colour 47 icons, even if the text specifically says 46.5%.

And be aware that more precise numbers (such as 47) will require the 100-icon grid. But to represent, say, 40%, you could use a grid of 100 or create a grid of 50 icons and colour 20. For that matter, you could even create 10 icons and colour 4! But don't try to show 47% using only 10 icons.

WAFFLE CHARTS

A useful variant of an icon array is a waffle chart, which is, in fact, a table!

Insert a slide with some white space for your data. Now insert a table that is ten by ten cells. This represents 100%. It's like a square pie!

On the table Layout tab, you'll need to adjust the overall table dimensions to form a square (15 cm by 15 cm, for example). Then select the table and click Distribute Rows and Distribute Columns on the Layout tab. Now all your cells are squares of the same size, and each cell represents 1%.

With all cells selected, format the waffle grid by changing the Pen Colour for the cell borders to the same colour as the slide background, and apply All Borders under **Table Design** > Borders. Add the data by selecting and filling the appropriate cells.

You can represent more than one data series in a waffle, as shown in Figure 16.15. As with a pie chart, don't try to show too much with a waffle chart, though. If you

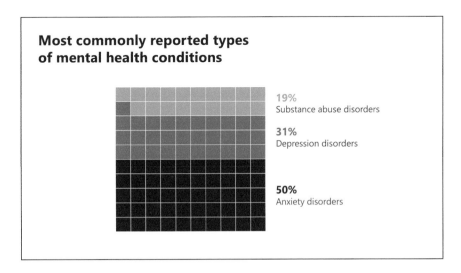

Figure 16.15 A waffle chart is just a table with square cells.

163

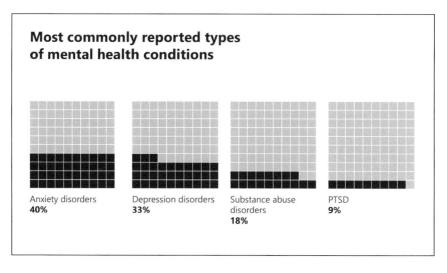

Most commonly reported types of mental health conditions

| Anxiety disorders | Depression disorders | Substance abuse disorders | PTSD |
| **40%** | **33%** | **18%** | **9%** |

Figure 16.16 An example of four smaller waffle charts, each with one data point.

need more than three data points, consider creating a single waffle for each, as you can see using the fictitious data in Figure 16.16.

HOW TO DETERMINE WHICH CHART TO USE

How do you choose the correct chart to best show your data? As you will have read above, the first question should be, "Do I really need a chart at all?". If you have decided that you do indeed need a chart, then consider which of the standard chart types is the best for your purposes.

You might also look online for inspiration. One guide we recommend is from The Visual Communication Guy[1]. Use the link below to find it, but please be sure to purchase the high-resolution version of the guide and don't just copy the image!

CONCLUSION

To present your data most successfully, consider your audience and think about your data. What is the main point, what do you want to focus on, and what's the best way to display the data? Break up the information if needed, leverage pre-attentive attributes, and focus on the key takeaways to make your charts and slides understandable at a glance. These things will help you tell the story of your data more effectively and get your point across more easily.

Further reading: Data visualisation is a hugely important topic, and we couldn't possibly cover as much detail in a single chapter as we would like. There are a number of excellent textbooks on the subject; here are some that we recommend (with thanks to Dr Gareth Lewis for help with putting this together).

Cole Nussbaumer Knaflic
Storytelling with data
Storytelling with data: Let's practice

Stephanie Evergreen
Effective data visualization
Presenting data effectively

Scott Berinato
Good charts
Good charts work-book

Stephen Few
Show me the numbers

Alberto Cairo
How charts lie
The truthful art

Bergstrom and West
Calling bullsh*t

Jon Schwabish
Better Data Visualizations

NOTE

1. https://thevisualcommunicationguy.com/2017/06/05/which-chart-should-i-use/

PART 4

Presenting

17

Teaching online using PowerPoint

"All changed, changed utterly: A terrible beauty is born".

Irish poet William Butler Yeates

We started planning this book in the early months of the COVID-19 pandemic. This pandemic changed the world of education in ways that were unimaginable before. A seminar room packed with eager learners was no longer the norm. As the pandemic eased, educators realised that face-to-face learning had some disadvantages. Staff on complex rotas or who lived at a distance could attend online sessions much more easily.

We have all heard masterful speakers who can keep an audience enthralled for an hour or more, but truthfully, these are rare. Most medics have experience with long, complex lectures where the audience struggle to maintain focus. Long, complex lectures online are even worse!

IN-PERSON TEACHING

The traditional in-person lecture is usually linear. The presenter proceeds through their slides in order, usually without interruption. These talks last up to an hour. Audience members falling asleep is not uncommon! In a hospital environment, audience members being paged/bleeped is normal, and this can be distracting for both the speaker and the audience.

On the other hand many of the supposed "new" concepts in online teaching are well-rehearsed with in-person sessions. For example, break-out rooms are a real rather than a virtual thing! Questions can be asked directly rather than electronically, although recently, social media has been used at conferences for questions.

DOI: 10.1201/9781003287902-21

ONLINE TEACHING

We have all used programmes such as Zoom™ or Microsoft Teams™ to screen share a live or pre-recorded presentation. This requires a new skill set to achieve best results.

The online audience can easily lose focus. They may be unable to see the presenter clearly; they are more likely to multitask, perhaps checking their email or social media.

Questions

Questions can be challenging because with multiple participants, it can be difficult to work out who is asking the question when participants cover several screens. Using the raised hand function is a useful way to resolve this. Alternatively, the chat function can be used for questions.

Keep it short(er)

Considering these issues, current thinking is that online presentations should be kept very short, ideally not over ten to fifteen minutes in length, or you could insert planned breaks in your longer presentation to allow the audience to refocus[1,2]. This is a good time to give the viewer's brain a chance to reset.

Remember Sweller's Cognitive Load Theory (Chapter 1). Breaking your presentation into digestible segments or introducing changes in style will help with information retention.

Interaction

It is worth breaking up longer sessions by using different styles of interaction to maintain attention. An interactive presentation that engages the audience in a two-way dialogue can suit small- to medium-sized audiences, whether in-person or online, but it can be more difficult to manage online.

Varying the styles of participant engagement might take the form of break-out rooms, panel discussions or simply questions both to and from audience members. Interactive presentations will work best if there is a moderator to handle questions in the chat function or to direct a panel. Interaction can be in the form of quizzes or polls. Interaction can also take the form of pre-course tasks, which are then presented to the group.

You might start with introductions and a poll such as: *What do you want to get out of this session?* Then provide a ten-minute talk, followed by discussion in breakout rooms. If you are teaching, try working through an explanation of the topic for ten minutes, then give the learners a task to complete either on their own or in breakout rooms, and then bring them together to work through their conclusions.

To get the best from online teaching, we suggest you focus on the following areas.

- Eye contact and hand gestures will help convey emotion, so keep your video feed on if you can. It may help to present standing up rather than seated.
- Use participants' names if possible. Give them a warning that a question is coming their way before you ask a question.
- Vary your tone, pitch and speed as you speak. Nothing is worse than a monotonous drawl.
- Include stories in your presentation. Obviously these must be relevant, but they help connect you with the audience.

SYNCHRONOUS LEARNING

Synchronous learning requires that the learner is present (online or in person) at the time of the teaching, which may not always be possible. Medical trainees may be geographically dispersed or may be unable to attend due to shift patterns. For the educator, online synchronous teaching can be challenging. They must master the technology and then deliver at a faster pace, which can inhibit interaction with students.

To make this work well, two trainers are ideal: One to handle the technology and one to provide the learning. Pre-recording your talk (Chapter 19) can take much of the stress out of synchronous online teaching. Showing a pre-recorded presentation means you don't have to narrate the talk, allowing you to concentrate on other tasks such as collating the questions coming in via the chat function.

ASYNCHRONOUS LEARNING

Traditionally Bloom's taxonomy places the classroom-based lecture at the base of the educational pyramid. In the "Flipped Classroom", much of the learning will be asynchronous, which means that the learners will view the teaching material in their own time from your pre-recorded presentations.

This takes much of the stress of synchronous teaching away from the educator but requires the educator to either access or learn how to record high-quality content. This model allows the learner more time to consider responses to questions and prepare their own queries, which will further enhance learning. In addition asynchronous learning allows trainees to choose when and where to do the pre-course reading or viewing, and the live sessions will be shorter.

The downside is that there are often multiple potential or real distractions in these new learning environments. Added to this it has been suggested that the attention span with online learning is very short, possibly less than ten minutes.

However some have challenged this, suggesting that attention span relates more to delivery style and content than any fixed length of talk. Whichever is true, it is likely that for online teaching, pre-recorded material must be focussed and videos generally shorter than the traditional lecture.

Students who have grown up with face-to-face teaching may be uncomfortable with this new way of working. We have found that some learners do not engage with the pre-course materials (even with multiple reminders), perhaps out of habit. Undoubtedly some trainers will find this new world daunting.

How to flip a classroom

To "Flip" the classroom, you would do the following[3]:

1. Create your videos using techniques like those shown in Chapter 18 or with your local audio-visual experts.
2. Notify the learners about the pre-course material and the importance of reading/viewing it.
3. Use the time for the live meeting wisely. The preparatory learning should allow better engagement in class. You should reduce the in-class "sit and listen" and increase the "do and learn".

DUAL MONITORS

It may also help to have an extended desktop or a second monitor when teaching online. This allows you to view and share your presentation on one screen and the chat feedback and questions on a second screen.

CONCLUSION

There is no doubt that medical education is changing rapidly. The bad old days when you could just type a few lines of text on your slides and then give a talk have gone.

Online teaching is the future, and the future is here now! A terrible beauty is born; let's emphasise the beauty and minimise the terrible!

NOTES

1. Balan, A.K.; Jacintos, A.R.; Montemayor, T. The Influence of Online Learning towards the Attention Span and Motivation of College Students. 2020. Available online: https://www.researchgate.net/publication/348916010_The_Influence_of_Online_Learning_towards_the_Attention_Span_and_Motivation_of_College_Students
2. Sobral K et al. Active methodologies association with online learning fatigue among medical students. *BMC Med Educ.* 2022; 22: 74.
3. https://www.walesdeanery.org/sites/default/files/How%20to%20Flip%20the%20Classroom.pdf

18

Present like the pros

Making an impression requires more than great slides. You want all elements of the presentation to go well, from when you stand up to speak until you sit back down again.

Think back to the last session that you were at. The speaker arrives at the podium and looks despairingly at the desktop of the computer, searching for their talk. You, meantime, are wondering what that other file on the desktop marked "Serious Adverse Incidents" is about! The hapless presenter finally finds the file and opens it in Normal View in PowerPoint. Your heart sinks as you see there are over 100 slides and it appears they are almost all text. As you are considering a coffee break, the presenter is now trying to persuade the mouse to hover over the tiny icon to start up their presentation.

After coffee, the next presenter is called up. They tap a single key on the keyboard and the first slide appears. Joy of joys, it is not a white slide with black text!

Which of these presenters do you think you will enjoy more? In this chapter we will talk through how you can learn to present like a pro.

APPEARANCE

How you dress may be important, depending on the situation. Obviously, for an in-house meeting, standard clothing or scrubs will suffice. However you may need to "dress to impress" for a more formal session.

As a general rule the more important the occasion, the more formally you should dress. These days a suit is rarely necessary, but a smart top and well-pressed trousers or a dress/skirt are a minimum. Make sure you polish your shoes and tidy your hair. If you wear jewellery, be sure that it doesn't rattle when you move.

If there's a chance that you'll use a lavalier mic, wear a belt or clothing the battery pack can clip to without causing wardrobe malfunctions. These little things can be annoying distractions.

DOI: 10.1201/9781003287902-22

PREPARATION AND BACKUP PLANS

Before your session starts be sure that your presentation is loaded on the computer and test it to make sure all is working as planned. This is especially vital if you are using video. It is always wise to have a backup plan should the technology fail—and it sometimes will!

If presenting in a setting where logging in is required, it is a good idea to email your talk to the person logging on for the session. This will save you from having to change users on the computer used for the session. Send a copy to your own email address just in case.

If you have a secure USB stick such as an IronKey™, keep a copy on that. Finally the ultimate backup is a PDF version of your talk. You can show PDF files just like PowerPoint, though there will be no animations.

If you are speaking in an unfamiliar setting, be sure to find out where your presentation file is on the computer, as well as how you control the sound level and the lights in the room. Don't wait until you are speaking to ask about this.

If you are hosting a meeting on your computer, tidy the desktop, removing all unnecessary files and moving the rest into folders so that the presentation files can be easily found. You can hide your desktop icons (Windows: Right-click on desktop > View > untick Show Desktop Icons; on a Mac there are several apps that you can download that do this), but before you hide the icons, place all your presentation files in an open folder so that they can be accessed easily.

REMOTE CONTROLS

If you are using a remote control (clicker), be sure it is connected and working. If you don't own the remote, do you know which button to press to advance the slides? Many remotes have a red laser pointer—be aware that this will not show up on a TV monitor. Some rooms will be set up so that laser pointers will be difficult to use; maybe the screen is far away or at an awkward angle to the presenter. So don't rely on a laser to point to specific things on your slides.

STARTING UP

When you arrive at the lectern, find your PowerPoint file. You have two options to start the presentation: If the file is open in Normal mode (as you would use it for editing), just hit F5 on Windows or ⌘-Return on a Mac and the presentation will start. Some Windows computers require Function-F5 to start the slide show.

These shortcuts avoid hunting around for the **Start Presentation** icon or going through the slide show menu items.

PowerPoint SHOW

You may want to try saving your presentation as a PowerPoint Show file (see Chapter 12); then you just double-click on the file to start the presentation in Slide Show view (and no one will see any of your other slide thumbnails) (Figure 18.1).

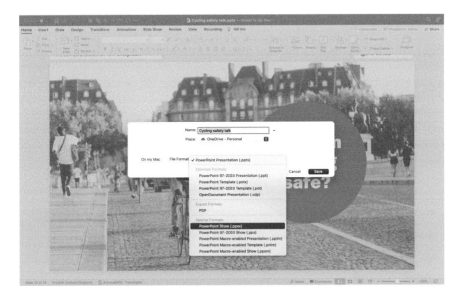

Figure 18.1 **Saving as a PPSX file.**

IF YOU ARE THE FIRST SPEAKER

A useful trick if you are speaking first is to get to the computer before the session, open your first slide in Slide Show mode, and then hit the B key. This will give you a black screen.

When you're ready to begin, hit B again, and the first slide will reappear. Alternatively use W for a white screen.

DELIVERY

Now it is time to start speaking.

You should have been practising so you know exactly what you will say. Slow down and take steady breaths. A common mistake is to speak far too fast.

Avoid fillers; words like "OK" or "em" are used to give you time to think about what to say next, often subconsciously. Indeed, many speakers habitually use these and are blissfully unaware that they do. You can practice your talk in front of a friend or colleague and ask them to look out for this.

Speaker Coach

In Microsoft 365, you can use the Speaker Coach to tell you about pace, fillers and other aspects of your talk that you may not be aware of. Start your presentation (granting access to your microphone if necessary) and just present as normal.

Figure 18.2 is a report from Speaker Coach for a presentation.

If you are speaking in a noisy environment or where the sound system is poor, think about using PowerPoint's built-in Closed Captioning. This can also translate your presentation into a choice from several languages with reasonable accuracy, which may be helpful to an audience where English is not their first language. Very few presenters are aware of this amazing AI built right into PowerPoint in Microsoft 365.

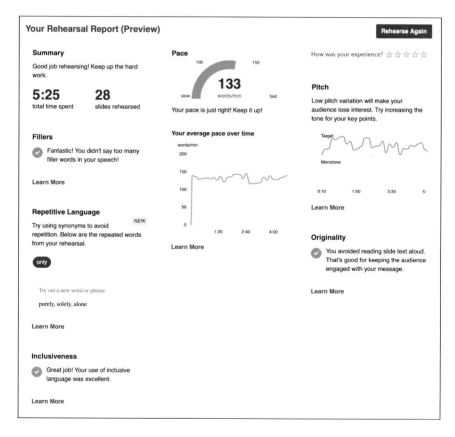

Figure 18.2 Speaker Coach.

To enable captions, select Always Use Subtitles in the **Slide Show** tab of the ribbon. You should select the spoken and subtitle languages in the Subtitles Settings menu, and you can change how your subtitles will appear there. Click More Settings (Windows) or System Caption Preferences (Mac) to further alter the caption styles.

CAMEO

Microsoft 365 has a new feature called Cameo. Cameo allows you to add a view of your camera feed as you present or record (see Chapter 19). You can access Cameo by using the **Insert** tab. If you are going to use Cameo, it is better to design your slides so that a space is available for the video feed; you don't want it overlapping your on-slide information, so plan ahead.

To activate your camera feed, click Camera Preview on the **Camera Format** tab of the ribbon. You can edit, resize, and reposition the Cameo object just like any shape. While there are lots of options for this, we suggest that you keep it simple. A circle or rectangle with unobtrusive edges is all that is needed.

Cameo might be useful if you are speaking in a very large venue, where the audience can't see your face clearly. Our colleague Chantal Bossé[1] has suggested an innovative use would be to attach another camera to your computer and use it to show someone signing during your presentation.

FINISHING

When you reach the end of your presentation, make sure it's clear you're finished (see Chapter 3).

QUESTIONS

You may be able to anticipate potential questions. If so, you can make slides specifically to answer these. This can be very effective but requires careful preparation. In anticipation of these questions, make slides at the end of your presentation exactly as normal. Right-click on these slides in the slide thumbnails and choose Hide Slide. The slide thumbnail will be greyed out and a universal prohibitory symbol (a circle with a diagonal line) will appear on the thumbnail. You can also hide and unhide slides on the **Slide Show** tab of the ribbon.

Now when someone asks you a question for which you have a pre-prepared slide, just type the slide number for that slide and then hit the Return key (Mac) or Enter (Windows).

You may want to finish your presentation with a black slide. If this is not happening by default, on a Mac go to PowerPoint > Preferences > Slide Show and click End with black slide (**File** > Options > Advanced > End with black slide on

Windows). You must keep either your final slide or this black slide on screen until all questions are finished. If you don't, you will exit Slide Show mode and cannot show the hidden slides without restarting the presentation.

Of course, you can go back to any slide using this technique. It is pretty slick to say, "Yes, I think you were referring to this table" and hit the number for the relevant slide and then Return (⌘) or Enter (Win) to show the table in question. You will need to know the slide numbers, so print off a handout showing all your slides.

USING PRESENTER VIEW BY DEFAULT

On a Mac when you open PowerPoint > Preferences > Slide Show the option "Always start Presenter View with two displays" is available to you. It is worth ensuring this is ticked so that when you connect to an external display, presenter view will start on your computer. Alternatively, you can use the Presenter View button on the **Slide Show** tab. On Windows, you just need to tick the box for Use Presenter View on the **Slide Show** tab (Figure 18.3).

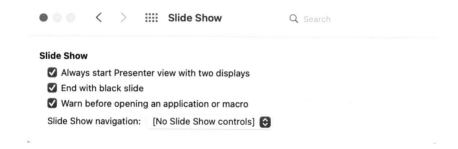

Figure 18.3 **Always start Presenter view with two displays (Mac).**

Presenter View allows you to see the current slide and the next slide. The thumbnails of your slides are shown at the bottom of the window on Mac. On Windows click the "See All Slides" grid button. The current time and the duration of your talk are also displayed. Notes can be typed and edited while using Presenter View (this is a new feature; if it doesn't work, you may need to update PowerPoint) or as you edit the slides in Normal View (the default editing view). You can also drag the edges of the panes to enlarge the speaker notes area or the next slide thumbnail, for example. If Presenter View is showing on the wrong monitor, use Swap Displays (Mac) or Display Settings > Swap Presenter View and Slide Show View (Windows) to switch it (Figures 18.4 and 18.5).

The notes in Presenter View are only seen on your computer. The audience will see a standard PowerPoint display.

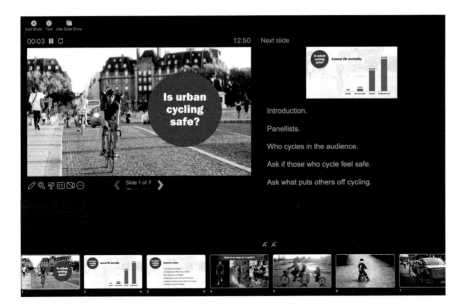

Figure 18.4 **Presenter view on a Mac.**

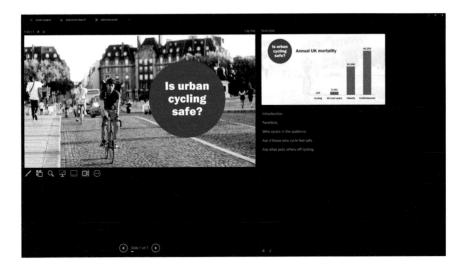

Figure 18.5 **Presenter view on Windows.**

SUMMARY

Hopefully this chapter will help less experienced presenters to hone their skills.

Think about the presentation journey. How will you dress? Do you know the room where you are presenting? Do you have a backup plan? Can you use some of the tips in this chapter to make the process look slick and professional? How will you finish your talk and how will you handle questions?

By planning all these elements, hopefully, your next presentation will wow your audience.

NOTE

1. Chantal Bossé is the author of Microsoft PowerPoint Best Practices, Tips, and Techniques.

19

Recording a presentation

Recording your presentation in PowerPoint specifically refers to recording yourself narrating your presentation. Your camera and audio feed will be captured and placed as a small video on each slide.

There are many advantages to pre-recording your PowerPoint presentation. You can be sure that you will cover everything that needs to be included. You can redo it until it is perfect. You can ensure it will fit within the allocated time slot. When you show it online, you can relax and observe the learners to see if they are engaged. You can watch the chat function for questions and prepare answers.

There are many hardware and software tools for recording teaching material, but these are mostly beyond the scope of this book. We will focus on how to record your PowerPoint presentations for online viewing.

SETTING UP

You will need a suitable room, ideally somewhere where there is not too much ambient noise. Choose a quiet time of day, free from interruptions. Switch your phone to silent and turn your Wi-Fi off to avoid alerts during your recording. Put a "do not disturb" sign on your door if there's a chance someone might ring the bell.

Next you need a computer with reasonable processing power. You don't want the computer fan furiously whirring in the background of your talk!

The computer microphone may be sufficient for recording your narration, but if you can afford it, buy a USB microphone and a pop filter to reduce plosives (the popping sound that accompanies "P's" in particular). The camera on your computer may be adequate for the task, but if you do a lot of recording, a higher-resolution USB webcam is worth considering. Some of these have a very good microphone built in.

DOI: 10.1201/9781003287902-23

Your video camera should sit at eye level, so you may want to raise the computer on a pile of books or a laptop stand. This avoids that unflattering "up the nose" look!

LIGHTING

Next you need to consider lighting. A simple desk light may be adequate, but avoid bright lights behind you, in the ceiling, or from one or other side. You should aim to illuminate your face without any one area being too bright, ideally with a little shadow to one side of your nose (the Rembrandt effect[1]).

TIDY UP!

Carefully look at the video feed before you start and avoid any potential distractions behind you. If you wear glasses, are they clean? Are you wearing patterned clothing, which can cause the Moiré effect on video?[2]

HOW LONG SHOULD YOUR RECORDING LAST?

There is a current opinion that learners learn best in short bursts, maybe as short as ten minutes. The evidence for this is incomplete[3], but it is known that a detailed, lengthy diatribe is not the ideal way to learn.

Either keep your talk short or ensure that there are breaks in the detailed learning that allow the learner to relax a little and process the information to date. Demonstrations, videos, questions and polls are great ways to break up a heavy session.

Make sure you have practised well before you start recording. You may want to record this in one or two takes—believe us, you probably won't achieve that, certainly not on the first few attempts!

THE CAMEO CAMERA OBJECT

As we are writing this book, Microsoft has begun to introduce a new camera object called Cameo, which lets you format and position your video feed on your slides while you're designing your presentation. On Mac, click **Recording** > Cameo and insert the video feed onto each slide. On Windows, use **Record** > Cameo and choose the option to insert on the selected slide or all slides. On both Mac and Windows, select the Cameo object on the slide and use the tools on the Camera Format tab to reshape or reformat the camera feed (Figures 19.1 and 19.2).

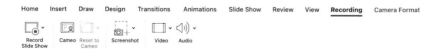

Figure 19.1 **Recording tab on Mac.**

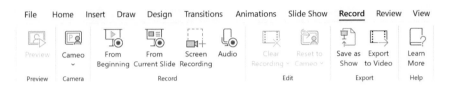

Figure 19.2 **Record tab on Windows.**

RECORDING YOUR PRESENTATION

Once you're ready to record (or practice recording!) your presentation, click **Recording** > From Beginning or From Current Slide. This opens the new Teleprompter View, which looks similar to Presenter View but is specifically designed to be used when recording narrations.

In Teleprompter View, click the camera icon to toggle your camera feed on and off in the Cameo object. (You may want audio but no video on selected slides.) Make sure your microphone is on as well. Click the arrows next to the camera and mic on the Mac to choose different options; on Windows, click the three dots (Figures 19.3 and 19.4).

Text that you have typed in the speaker notes area in Normal view will appear here for you to refer to as you're recording. You may want to enable automatic scrolling for your notes, which will begin when you start recording. (If you plan

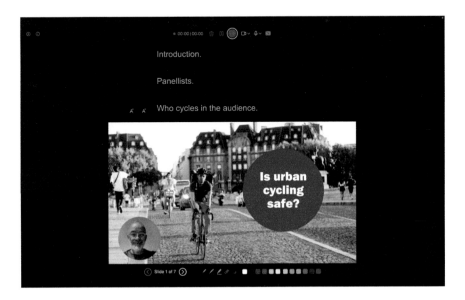

Figure 19.3 **Teleprompter view on Mac.**

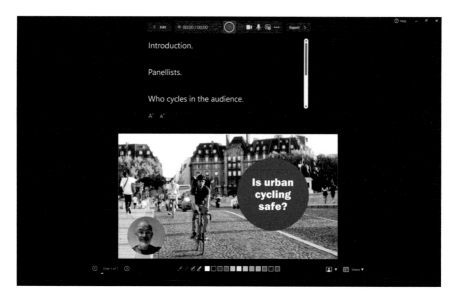

Figure 19.4 Teleprompter view on Windows.

to use auto-scroll, it's worth doing a practice recording so you can adjust the speed of the notes to your liking.) There is also a timer at the top of the screen; on the left is the time on the current slide and to the right is the total recording time.

You'll be able to pause and restart the recording at any time. Don't worry that you are looking at Teleprompter View; the recording is of the Slide Show View as normal.

Click the big red Record button in Teleprompter View to start recording your presentation. Advance through the slides as you normally would—using the spacebar, a clicker, or even the next slide arrow in Teleprompter View. Use the pens to annotate and draw on the slide image in Teleprompter View; identical markings will appear on the recorded Slide Show View as well. When you're finished, click the red button to stop recording.

Reviewing your recordings

Preview the recordings by clicking the Play button that appears on each slide image in Teleprompter View after you've recorded.

Exiting Teleprompter View saves the Cameo object as a video of you talking during that slide. It also saves transition timings based on the length of time you recorded and sets the transition to occur automatically.

184

REDOING A RECORDING

If you are unhappy with your recording, go back to the **Recording** tab and click Record Slide Show to re-open Teleprompter View. Advance to the slide you want to re-record. Click the bin button (Mac) or the Retake Recording button (Windows) to delete the existing recording for that slide.

You can now re-record the narration for that slide. If you do re-record a single slide, just stop recording and don't move on to the next slide when you are finished. Otherwise, your new recording will overwrite the existing recording on the next slide.

You can also clear the recordings from the **Recording/Record** tab. Clear will remove the camera object altogether from your slide. You can also choose Reset Cameo Object, which will remove your recorded narration but which will leave the empty Cameo object in place.

You cannot delete the video feed and retain the audio on individual slides. However, if you want sound without a video on a particular slide, simply drag the video window off the edge of the slide.

Once you are happy with the narration for your presentation, save the file, which now includes the audio and video (camera feed) recordings and automatic transition timings. You can always go back later and change one or more slide recordings. However, if the set-up in your recording space is not identical, the audio may be noticeably different.

TIPS FOR RECORDING

Go through your slides as if you were presenting to an audience. Remember to keep up a reasonable tempo and vary your pitch. Try to be engaging, even though there is no one to engage with! This is much easier if you are in a quiet room on your own. It may help to present standing up. This can improve the pitch and tempo, which will help add emotion to your delivery.

In Chapter 18, we mentioned using Speaker Coach to help you avoid filler words and to check your pace and pitch. Of course, do this before you actually start recording!

Silently count to five before you begin to leave a bit of wiggle room when you fire up the completed presentation with recorded narrations. We'll elaborate on this later.

A word of warning about transitions

Your narration is recorded and embedded in each slide in your deck. If you speak during the slide transitions, that part of your narration will not be recorded, so be careful to finish speaking before you transition to the next slide. For this reason, it is best to keep slide transitions at or below 0.7 seconds. (Check the transition duration for each slide in the Transitions tab of the ribbon.)

When you have finished your last slide pause for a few seconds, then stop recording as described above.

SAVING YOUR RECORDING

PowerPoint presentation (.pptx)

Save your talk as you learnt in Chapter 12 as a .pptx file.

You can open this file and play the slide show just as with any PowerPoint presentation. Once you're in Slide Show View, PowerPoint will play your narration and advance the slides for you. You can sit back and relax.

Why did we recommend a pause of five seconds at the start of your talk?

If you are screen sharing the recorded presentation, you may want to open PowerPoint, start your presentation (remember that's F5 on a PC and ⌘ + Return on a Mac), and immediately hit the B key on your keyboard. That will pause your presentation and show a black slide. When you are ready to begin the screen share, you need only hit B again to start—everything is set up and ready to go. If you prefer a white screen, hit the W key instead. Pausing for five seconds before recording gives you time to pause the presentation after putting it into Slide Show view so your narration doesn't start prematurely.

PowerPoint Show (.ppsx)

You may want to save your talk as a PowerPoint Show, which, as you know, opens the presentation directly in Slide Show View. You can do this from the **Record** tab in Windows or Mac using the typical Save As process. If you need to review how to do this, see Chapter 12.

If you are sending PPSX or PPTX files to others, the recipient will need to have PowerPoint on their computer or iPad to see these presentations. They can also view the presentation online in a browser if they have a (free) Microsoft account.

Video

You can also export your recorded presentation as a video. On a Mac go to **File** > Export, and from the File Format options, select MP4. On Windows you can use **Record** > Export to Video, or you can use **File** > Export > Create a Video. The MP4 video file format is cross-platform compatible so that it will play on a Mac or on Windows.

Video files are suitable for uploading to sites like YouTube™ or Learning Management Systems. The viewer does not need PowerPoint on their computer or tablet to watch the video.

Note: If you will use Zoom to show your pre-recorded MP4 file, click the Share Screen button in Zoom and then select the Advanced tab and click the Video button. This will automatically enable the options to Share sound and Optimise for video clips, which will greatly improve the quality of the video and audio feed.

THIRD PARTY SOFTWARE

You can create a freer-flowing presentation using third-party software; our preference is Camtasia. This is because it avoids the need to pause your speech between slides. You can also add more professional video effects, such as poster frames and crossfades between slides and sections of your talk. If you are likely to make lots of presentation videos, it is worth exploring software such as OBS Studio (which is free) or Camtasia. Camtasia does offer an educational discount.

SUMMARY

Recording your slide show in advance is a great way to make your presentation look professional while freeing you up as you show it. This means you can relax and watch your audience or the chat function if you are screensharing. It has the added advantage of ensuring that you keep to time.

Learners will appreciate your recordings, especially if you can make them accessible on demand. It takes practice to get the recordings right—but rest assured, it is worth it.

NOTES

1. https://en.wikipedia.org/wiki/Rembrandt_lighting
2. https://en.wikipedia.org/wiki/Moir%C3%A9_pattern
3. The Truth about Decreasing Attention Spans in University Students. https://tinyurl.com/2rfx3zvc

20

Creating useful handouts

There is no such thing as a great presentation that also works as a great handout—or is there? If you place everything you will say as text on your slides, that might work as a handout, but it will be a terrible presentation. If you create a stunning, visually appealing presentation, a handout of these slides will be meaningless, especially for the students who couldn't attend your lecture. In this chapter we show you how to create a handout that works well with a beautifully crafted, image-rich presentation.

POWERPOINT HANDOUTS

PowerPoint actually has a print option called handouts, and you can choose to print 1, 2, 3, 4, 6 or 9 slide thumbnails per page. You can use them as an aide memoir to assist you as you speak, but usually, giving them out isn't super helpful because the images are small (and unfortunately cannot be resized). PowerPoint handouts just don't cut it as a truly useful handout.

CREATING NOTES PAGES FOR YOURSELF

PowerPoint Notes Pages usually make better handouts than PowerPoint handouts do!

Notes Pages are designed to hold your speaker notes. As we explained in an earlier chapter, it's helpful to pull information into the speaker notes area (which is below the slide in Normal view) so you can streamline the text on your slides and make them more visual (Figure 20.1).

As you know, these speaker notes will appear in Presenter View, but you can also use Notes Pages to print them. To see what your notes pages will look like when printed, use **View** > Notes Pages. There should be a large slide thumbnail with the speaker notes below. You can resize and reposition the slide thumbnail and text placeholder. You can also edit, resize, and format the text by applying bold, italics, colour or highlights. Do be aware that while this type of formatting will appear in print or PDF, only bold, italics and underlines will display in Presenter View and Normal View (Figure 20.2).

DOI: 10.1201/9781003287902-24

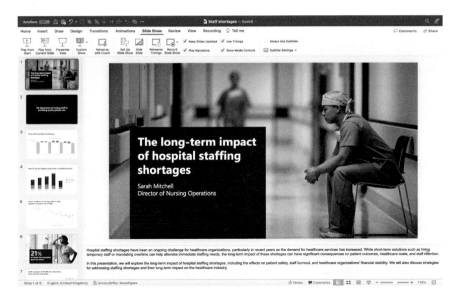

Figure 20.1 Speaker notes appear in the notes area below the slide.

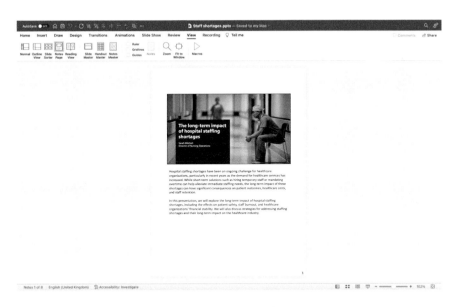

Figure 20.2 Notes page view.

You can print or create a PDF of your notes pages to refer to as you're speaking, or you could distribute these simple Notes Pages to others as a handout.

On a Mac go to **File** > Print, be sure the Layout is set to Notes, set the page layout to portrait under orientation as shown in Figure 20.3 and then select PDF > Save as PDF.

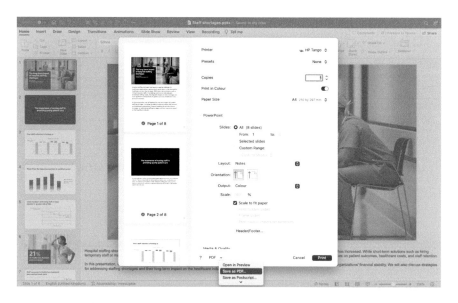

Figure 20.3 The save as PDF dialogue on a Mac.

On Windows, click **File** > Export > Create PDF/XPS Document > Create PDF/ XPS, and then be sure to click the Options button before you hit Publish. Choose Notes Pages from the Publish dropdown, and then OK and click Publish (Figure 20.4).

CREATING LEAVE-BEHINDS FOR OTHERS

Now that you understand the gist of creating and printing notes pages, you can leverage them to create handouts for others. The obvious drawback to using notes pages for handouts is that you might not want to give your speaker notes away as part of the handout! But with a little (simple) trickery, you can use the Notes feature to craft a great handout.

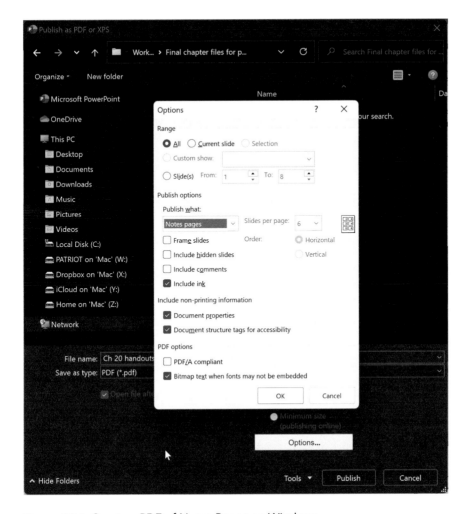

Figure 20.4 Create a PDF of Notes Pages on Windows.

Format the Notes Master

Start by opening the Notes Master from the **View** tab. Be careful and do not select Notes Page or Slide Master. You want to set up the Notes Master so you don't have to format the notes page for every single slide (Figure 20.5).

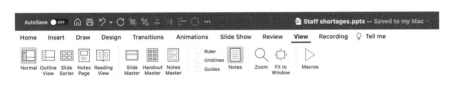

Figure 20.5 The View tab.

191

You will see a placeholder for headers and date at the top of the page and for footer and page number at the bottom. You probably only need the page number. You can delete the placeholders, you don't need or untick the boxes for header, date and footer in the Notes Master tab of the ribbon.

The Slide Image placeholder is, as the name suggests, where your slide thumbnail will appear. You clearly need this. Resizing and repositioning the Slide Image won't affect your presentation, just the handout you are about to create.

Below the slide image is a placeholder that contains five levels of text bullets. This is called the Body placeholder, and it holds the speaker notes you added in the Notes area either in Normal View or Presenter View. You want to keep this placeholder so you can see your notes in Presentation View, but you don't want these notes to appear in your handout. To achieve this, click on the edge of the body placeholder and drag it off the side of the page. That's the magic that makes this work! Your presenter notes are still available but won't be printed on your handout.

Finish formatting the Notes Master similarly to formatting a Slide Master. You may want to apply the same colour and font theme your slides use. You may also want to add some graphics to the page or a logo in a corner.

When you're done, click Close Master in the Notes Master tab and review your first slide in Normal View. You might want to confirm that you can still see your speaker notes in the notes area at the bottom of the screen!

Create a Notes Page for each slide

Now that you've set up the Notes Master, you can use the notes pages to create handouts for your slides. As explained above, choose **View** > Notes Page to open the notes page associated with the selected slide.

Instead of your speaker notes, you'll have lots of blank space below the slide image to add text boxes, charts, tables, images, or links. Just add whatever you need the same way as you would in a normal PowerPoint slide. The only difference is that this will be a page-sized document so that the font can be as small as 10 points, with no worries about legibility.

Be sure to format the text so that it looks professional. You should keep the text left aligned. Use the guides, SmartGuides, and Align tools to align the edges of your text boxes and images, just as you would on your slides (Figure 20.6).

The beauty of this is that the notes page is "attached" to the slide, so you'll have a ready-made handout page that is automatically included whenever you copy this slide into another file.

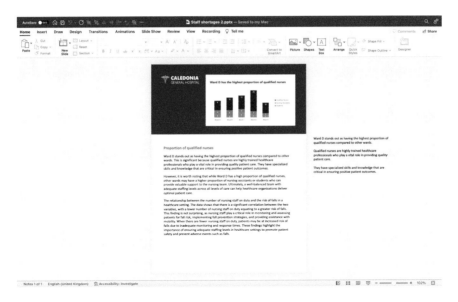

Figure 20.6 Completed notes page with body placeholder for speaker notes on the pasteboard and the handout text below the slide.

Create a PDF of the Notes Pages as described above. This PDF document can be emailed to the learners at the end of your talk. If your PDF is large, use WeCompress or NXPowerLite Desktop[1] to compress it and reduce the file size. If your handout is complex, it may exceed the email limit so that compression will be vital.

CONCLUSION

Learners will appreciate a good quality handout, especially those unable to attend your presentation. If you give a talk regularly, it is worth spending time on this. As you have seen in this chapter, crafting a handout is not difficult.

NOTE

1. https://neuxpower.com/nxpowerlite-desktop

21

Posters and visual abstracts

For many trainees a poster at a local meeting is their first foray into presenting audit or research projects. In the case of research scientists posters are an excellent way to present work before finalising it for publication. For others, posters are a great way to dip a toe in the river of scientific presentation, and let's be honest, they are a relatively painless way to enrich a portfolio.

However the experience for many poster authors is frequently underwhelming. Why do so few people stop to chat about your poster, the one that took you weeks to prepare and cost a fortune to print?

The answer is most likely the poster design, not the research. Poster viewers will skim posters to choose the ones to stop at. Those that are visually appealing, short, interesting, relevant and with a clear message will reel in the casual passer-by.

It's tempting to copy a previous poster layout. This may result in a boring series of posters, or worse, the same mistakes being repeated over and over. On the other hand once your department has a great poster layout, you can reuse it over and over.

In research for this book we learned the sad truth that few medics have received meaningful training in how to prepare a poster. In this chapter we will take you through the process. We will help you design an eye-catching poster and discuss how to develop an e-poster. Finally we will briefly touch on the preparation of a visual abstract.

We hope that meeting hosts might pay attention to this chapter because we have an important message for them at the end!

REMEMBER, IT'S A STORY NOT A SAGA!

Throughout this book we have emphasised that an engaging presentation contains as little text as possible. Many researchers think a poster is the opposite;

DOI: 10.1201/9781003287902-25

they must cram every aspect of their research onto it. This makes for a visually unappealing poster. Remember that the target is for the viewer to "get the message" at a glance.

A well-designed poster will draw attention and stop people walking by. This means minimal information is displayed as efficiently as possible. No one wants to stop at a poster and then have to work hard to understand it, so keep the message engaging and simple.

You will normally stand next to your poster during judging or be online for your virtual poster, so you can tell the story and fill in the gaps. You can direct the reader to further material using QR codes.

RTFM, OR IN GENTLER LANGUAGE, "READ THE INSTRUCTIONS"

Every meeting should have clear instructions for poster submission. In our research, we have found the quality of these instructions to vary enormously. Read the instructions and follow them diligently. They should at the very least set out the size and orientation (portrait or landscape) of the poster. Printers will have instructions on file type, usually requiring that you submit a PDF file.

Some meetings show posters on-screen; these e-posters are essentially a single slide presentation. These can be submitted as a .pptx or a .pdf file; the meeting instructions should specify this.

The organiser may specify that you cannot include industry logos and whether you should include the meeting/organisation logo.

There may also be instructions on acceptable methods of securing your poster (drawing pins are not great as they damage the poster; Blue Tack™ or Velcro™ are better).

SIZE MATTERS

We cannot emphasise this enough; you must design your poster to the dimensions required by the meeting organiser.

The most common size for poster submission is A0. Of course they do things differently in the US, where 48 by 36 inches is a common size. If you design your poster in a smaller size than this and include images which are not scalable (such as JPEGs), when you enlarge your file, these images will lose quality.

In the past some posters were produced as six A4 sheets, which were then stacked together to form a single poster. Don't do this. It may be easier to transport, but it looks amateurish.

SETTING THE PAGE SIZE IN PowerPoint

You can set your page size from the **Design** tab using Slide Size > Page Set Up.

If you want to change between centimetres (metric) and inches (US), this change is made in your operating system, not in PowerPoint. A quick Google search will show you how to do this.

For a landscape A0 poster, enter a horizontal dimension of 118.8 cm and a vertical dimension of 84.1 cm. When you choose OK, you will be warned that you are scaling up your page size. Click Scale and then OK on a Mac. In Windows, choose Ensure Fit.

The largest page size you can set in PowerPoint is 142.24 cm (56 inches). If your poster must be larger than this, halve the dimensions and choose print at 200% when printing.

Remember to save your presentation with an appropriate name, and as you continue your design, save again at regular intervals (or ensure that Autosave is switched on—see Chapter 12).

ESTABLISHING A "NO-FLY ZONE"

Forgive the military analogy but you will want to establish a "no-fly zone" around the edge of the poster. This is a safe area where there is no significant content. This avoids the risk of text being too tight to the edge or, worse, getting cut off during printing. A little white space around the edges gives everything breathing room and also makes the poster more visually appealing. We use guides to indicate these margins.

We recommend adding these guides at the master level. This prevents them from being inadvertently selected and moved while you work on the slide. Choose **View** > Slide Master and select the Blank Layout.

On the **View** tab, tick the box next to Guides to turn them on. You'll see two guides, one vertical and one horizontal, each centred on the slide. You can change the colour of any guide by right-clicking and choosing a new colour from the flyout menu.

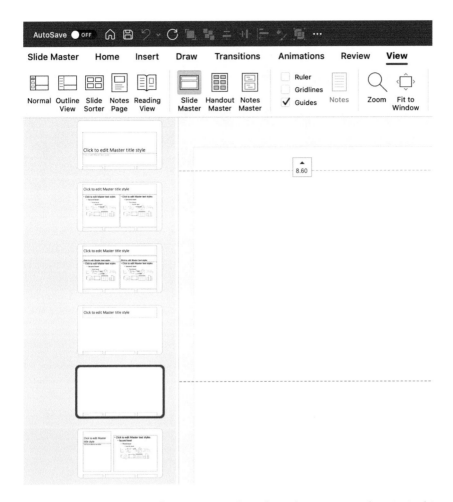

Figure 21.1 The position of the horizontal guide is shown as you drag it; in this case, 8.6 cm.

Right-click in an empty space on the slide (or off the slide altogether) and choose Grid and Guides > Horizontal Guide to add a new guide. Drag this new horizontal guide near the top of your slide and position it at 8.6 cm (see Figure 21.1). Now right-click, add another horizontal guide and drag it to the bottom of the slide area, stopping at 8.6 cm. The positions we've provided are just suggestions for the A0 poster size. Adjust as needed for your content and other poster sizes.

Following the same steps, add two vertical guides for the left and right margins. Position these vertical guides at 16.00 cm on the left and right sides of the slide area. The completed guide setup is shown in Figures 21.2 and 21.3.

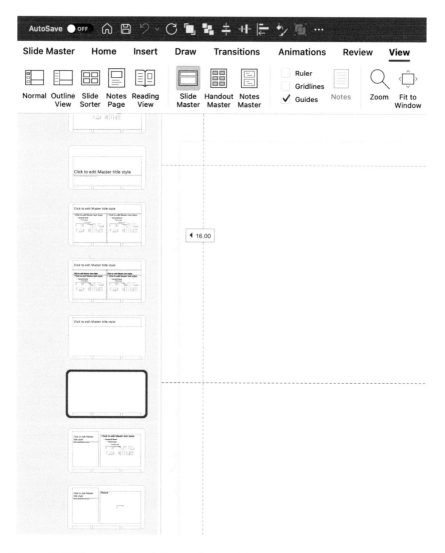

Figure 21.2 The position of the vertical guides.

Setting up columns

The most effective poster designs are neatly arranged and organised with the use of columns. You could define three, four or possibly more columns on your poster depending on the content to be included For this example we'll use guides to define four columns on the Blank layout.

We want the guides spaced evenly across the slide in between our new margins. It's easy to set this up using rectangles as temporary spacers. Draw a new rectangle

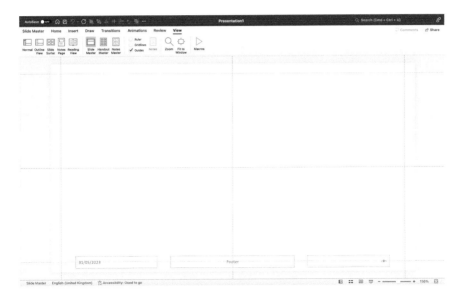

Figure 21.3 The blank layout in the Slide Master tab with four guides added to define margins. The blue guides are the default midline guides.

on the Blank layout and change the width to 7.5 cm. (This rectangle width is a suggestion based on an A0-sized poster. Adjust as you see fit.) Position the left edge of the rectangle so that it's aligned with the left margin guide. Duplicate the rectangle and move it slightly to the right. Repeat two times until you have four rectangles in a row. Align the right edge of the last rectangle with the right margin guide.

Finally, select the four rectangles and then **Align** > Distribute Horizontally to evenly space them across the slide. Refer to Chapter 9 if you need a refresher on distributing objects.

Right-click on a blank area of the slide, select Grid and Guides > Add a Vertical Guide. Position the guide on the right side of the first rectangle. Repeat adding vertical guides and positioning them on the left and right sides of the remaining rectangles. Now that all four columns are defined with guides you can delete the rectangles (Figure 21.4).

When setting up columns for other poster sizes, you can use a group of rectangles as temporary spacers. Draw a rectangle at approximate column width. Duplicate the rectangle for the number of columns on your poster, keeping a bit of space in between. Select the rectangles, **Align** > Distribute Horizontally, and then group them together. Position the left edge of the group to meet the left margin guide and stretch the right side of the group to meet the right margin guide. Add guides

Figure 21.4 The temporary rectangles used to correctly position the vertical guides.

on the left and right sides of the spacer rectangles to define poster columns and then delete the rectangles.

Close Master View to return to Normal View. We'll construct the poster on a blank slide. On the **Home** tab, press the Layout button and choose Blank.

LOGO POSITIONING

Review the meeting instructions regarding the use of logos. If you have a sponsor, are industry logos allowed? Is your work on behalf of a university or within a hospital or trust? If so, you may wish to include a logo.

Try to find a high-resolution version of your logo, download it to a folder and then insert it. You want an image of sufficient resolution that will not pixelate when placed on your poster.

Ideally these images should be vector images such as .svg, which can be scaled with no loss of quality. If you cannot get a vector image, use a raster image such as a .jpg or .png file, but be careful not to distort the logo. In the **Picture Format** tab on Mac, make sure that with the logo selected, the Lock Aspect Ratio box is ticked to the right of the logo dimensions. On Windows, you'll need to press and hold the Shift key while dragging a corner of the logo to resize.

Something we see quite often in posters is .jpeg logos with white backgrounds sitting atop coloured title areas. This isn't a good look! If you can get a logo with a transparent background (such as a .png), use that instead. If you cannot get a logo with a transparent background, then place the logo on a white area of the

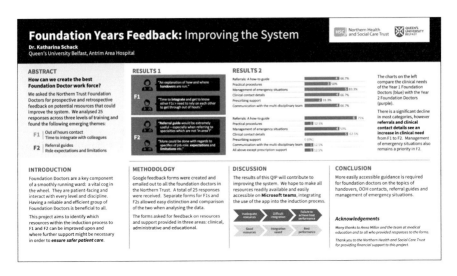

Figure 21.5 Our final poster was modified from the original with the author's permission. (Author: Dr Katharina Schack.)

poster. Have a look at Figure 21.3. The two logos are JPEGs and have been placed on top of a white box for this reason.

For our poster we continued to fill the text boxes as shown in Figure 21.5. The chart has been constructed using the principles outlined in Chapter 16.

COLOUR

Too much colour on a poster looks garish and should be avoided, but no one wants to look at a black-and-white poster. Try to limit the number of colours and choose colours that complement each other. In our poster (Figure 21.5) you see that colours have been re-used throughout.

PREPARING YOUR CONTENT

You will have submitted an abstract before your poster was accepted. It is important that the content of the poster reflects the content of the abstract. Open the abstract in a Word document.

The poster will need to be divided into sections, usually matching the standard scientific order of Background, Aims, Methods, Results, Discussion and References; although, in some instances these headings may vary. For example, you may include Acknowledgements and contact details.

Let's assume that you are using five headings. In addition, you will probably include some visual elements (charts, tables, or images).

Now divide the elements so that they will fit within your four columns. Don't produce long blocky columns; instead set up small text boxes with a few lines in each. These are much easier to read. You may find that sketching out your layout on paper first helps with this process.

One Big Idea, again!

Remember that concept of the "One Big Idea" we mentioned in Chapter 1? Where do you think is the best place to put your One Big Idea? Where do people look first?

Your title will be the first (and maybe last) bit of the poster that people will read. Use it to shout out that "One Big Idea".

Look at these titles for the same study; which poster would you stop at?

1. Consultants holding pagers and bleeps and filtering calls during unit-based teaching; can it reduce the interruptions to scheduled postgraduate teaching on a surgical unit?
2. A simple method to achieve bleep-free teaching.

Even if your research is on some obscure topic with long, hard-to-understand terminology, write the title in plain English so that a non-expert will understand it and stop to learn more.

Your title needs to shout your message loud and clear. Insert a text box in the top left corner of your poster and add a title that will grab attention. Consider an active title or a call to action rather than a boring description of the study.

Adding additional content

Your abstract is important, so you may want to format it differently from the rest of the poster. We used a different background in our example.

Left-aligned text is the best choice. Justified text is hard to read and creates a "wall of text" effect nobody wants to read.

If you use bulleted text please make sure the hanging indents are properly indented (see Chapter 6). This makes it easier to read.

Your methods and results section can consist of short notes or even (yes!) bullet points. Use charts and graphs as much as you can but use the techniques in the data visualisation chapter to make sure the message is clear.

Using QR codes

QR (Quick Response) codes are a great way to connect with a poster viewer. You can use the QR code to link to full publications, guidelines, videos and websites.

Alternative designs for your poster

Some poster designers suggest putting the study background text in the left column of the poster, the results and any charts or tables on the right, and the main message in the centre in large bold type. This is because you will likely stand to the right side and can discuss your poster with a viewer from there. A second person coming to your poster can stand on the left and read all about your study. The large central portion is where you place the "bait". This is where your catchy title or "One Big Idea" sits.

Printing your poster

You will need to identify a printer that is able to print posters; most universities have details of companies that can do this. You can also ask the printer if they have preferences for how you set up the PDF.

Save your poster as a PowerPoint file in the usual way as a backup. Now export it as a PDF as outlined in Chapter 12. That file can be emailed to the printer.

DESIGNING AN E-POSTER

An e-poster is shown on a computer screen rather than being printed out. Again you will need to read the conference instructions carefully. If you are presenting virtually—that is, sharing your computer screen—you will usually set the page size to Widescreen 16:9 just like any presentation.

If the poster is to be displayed on a monitor with you physically present, you need to know the aspect ratio of the monitor and whether the monitor is configured in landscape mode or portrait mode. If you cannot get information on the dimensions, it's usually safe to assume 16:9 (landscape) or 9:16 (portrait).

For landscape mode, just set up your page size as widescreen. If the meeting will display your e-poster in portrait mode, you need to change your page setup to reflect this. Go to **Design** > Slide Size > Custom Slide Size and select Slide Sized For Widescreen. Choose the portrait orientation, which is the top left icon on Mac. Click OK and then Scale Up (Mac) or choose Ensure Fit (Windows) (Figure 21.6).

Now you can follow the instructions above to set up safe zones at the edge of the slides and the number of columns you require.

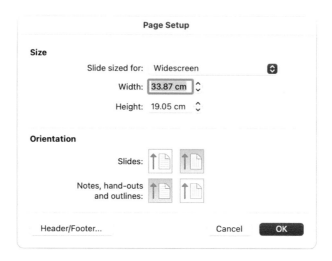

Figure 21.6 **Page Setup on a Mac.**

Submitting your e-poster

The meeting organiser will usually give clear instructions about the file format for e-posters. They may request a PowerPoint file, usually .pptx. If they require a PDF file, create one as previously described. This file can then be emailed to the conference.

A FEW THOUGHTS FOR MEETING ORGANISERS!

Many of the poster presenters that we interviewed for this chapter found poster instructions confusing. One recounted instruction to produce a portrait poster, only to find it projected on a landscape monitor, meaning that only half of the poster could be seen at one time.

In the instructions for presenters of physical posters, you should state the poster size (we recommend A0) and the orientation. You may wish to include some rules, especially regarding the inclusion of commercial logos and whether the conference logo should be included. Our view is that this should *not* be required—your conference logo will likely be visible all around the venue; let the poster reflect the topic under discussion.

It may be helpful to describe minimum text sizes for the title and content.

If e-posters are being submitted specify the monitor aspect ratio and orientation.

We have seen poster "templates" that submissions must adhere to. These were universally terrible! If you really must have a template, please ask a professional to design it.

DESIGNING A VISUAL ABSTRACT

WHAT IS A VISUAL ABSTRACT?

A visual abstract is a graphical representation of key information from a publication or presentation. Their purpose is to summarise the information with the minimum use of text so that viewers can understand the key messages at a glance.

Visual abstracts may look a little like posters, but they are designed for very different purposes and the two must not be confused. A visual abstract should encourage the viewer to read further, usually by seeking the related publication. They are ideally suited to dissemination on social media.

WHY PRODUCE A VISUAL ABSTRACT?

When your paper is accepted for publication the editor may request a visual abstract. Alternatively, you may feel that your paper can be enhanced by including a visual abstract, which may even tip the balance in favour of acceptance by the journal.

Of course, a visual abstract is a great way to disseminate the results of your work and will encourage readers to dive deeper and read the full paper.

The good news is that if you have read this book, you have the skills to create a basic visual abstract using PowerPoint. Of course, we would recommend using a professional designer if you can.

Setting up your visual abstract slide

As with a poster, you should start by choosing an appropriate size for your slide. Usually widescreen 16:9 (which should be your default) is perfect. Set safe margins as you learned earlier in this chapter.

Use as little text as you can, avoiding full sentences. Use icons to assist the viewer where possible (see Chapter 7). Simple two-dimensional icons are preferable to colourful or 3D icons. Make sure they show diversity—avoid inappropriate gender or racial icons.

Place your text in text boxes, left aligned and using a legible font. Don't underline text; it adds visual clutter and can look like a link. You should use the same font throughout, but you can vary font size and colour to emphasise information. Be conscious of the alignment and spacing of text and icons. Using guides might be helpful as you lay things out.

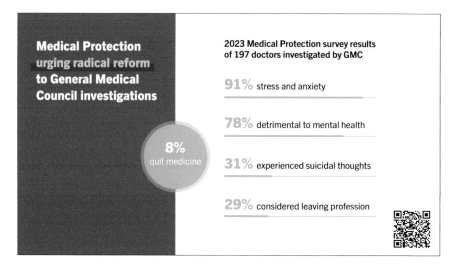

Figure 21.7 A visual abstract based on a detailed report with a QR code link to the report. (Used with permission from the Medical Protection Society.)

Don't cut and paste charts and graphs from your paper or presentation into the visual abstract; they will be tiny and hard to read. Instead, look for better visualisation techniques which summarise your points.

Don't be afraid to leave white space; this makes the information easier to read (Figure 21.7).

CONCLUSION

Posters are really only big slides! They are a great way to learn many of the techniques laid out in this book and a great place to finish!

Index

Note: Page numbers refer to text and those in *italic* refer to figures.